NEVER BE AFRAID TO DO THE RIGHT THING

*A Leadership Guide
in an Age of Change
and Challenge*

Gerald S. Levey, MD

Dean Emeritus

David Geffen School of Medicine at UCLA

**The Lincy Foundation
Distinguished Service Chair**

Distinguished Professor of Medicine

SECOND RIVER
HEALTHCARE PRESS

Bozeman, Montana

NEVER BE AFRAID TO DO THE
RIGHT THING

*A Leadership Guide in an Age
of Change and Challenge*

Second River Healthcare Press
26 Shawnee Way,
Suite C
Bozeman, MT 59715

Phone (406) 586-8775
FAX (406) 586-5672

Editor: Tiffany Young
Cover Design: Lan Weisberger — Design Solutions
Typesetting/Composition: Neuhaus/Tyrrell Graphic Design

Levey, Gerald
Never be Afraid to Do the Right Thing / Gerald S. Levey, MD

ISBN-13: 978-1-936406-07-4 (hard cover)   ISBN-13: 978-1-936406-08-1 (soft cover)
ISBN-13: 978-1-936406-09-8 (E-Book)

1. Health services administration.   2. Leadership.   3. Inspiration.

Library of Congress Control Number: 2011924667

First Printing   August 2011

Second River Healthcare Press books are available at special quantity discounts. Please call for information: (406) 586-8775 or order from the website: **www.SecondRiverHealthcare.com** or **www.NeverBeAfraidToDoThe RightThing.com**

CONTENTS

Publisher's Page   ii

Table of Contents   iii

Praise For *Never Be Afraid to Do the Right Thing*   v

About the Book   xvii

Foreword   xix

Preface   xxiii

Dedication   xxix

Acknowledgements   xxxi

1. **The Shaping of a Future Leader**   1
2. **Academic Health Centers**   13
3. **Primer for Aspiring Leaders**   23
4. **The First Faculty Meeting and The First Year**   41
5. **"Good Morning, How Are You Today?"**   49
6. **Decisions, Decisions, Decisions**   57
7. **Financial Management**   71
8. **The Vision, The Mission and The Strategic Plan**   79
9. **Recruitment and Retention**   89
10. **Mentoring**   95
11. **Governance Boards**   107
12. **Advice for Search Committees**   113
13. **Crisis Management**   121
14. **Fund-Raising**   137
15. **Every Leader Needs a Joke**   157
16. **I'd Do It Again**   181

Appendix   189

Bibliography   205

About the Author   207

NEVER BE AFRAID TO DO THE RIGHT THING

Jerry Levey is known as the dean of medical school deans. During his long and illustrious term as vice chancellor of Health Sciences and dean of the Geffen School of Medicine at UCLA, he built one of the world's premier academic health centers. Jerry is known for his scholarship, humanity and ethics. I have personally benefited from Jerry's knowledge and generosity. When I returned to UC San Diego to be dean, Jerry was the first one to call and offer me congratulations (and condolences). Since then, he has been my guide through the byzantine administration of the University of California, and he continues to give me invaluable thoughtful advice.

It is not surprising that Jerry's new book is articulate, thoughtful, engaging, witty and funny, just as Jerry is. This book provides a coherent approach to leadership in American academic health centers, written by someone who has seen it all, done it all and lived to tell about it. The book provides insightful discussions on key areas of strategic planning, mentoring and governance. But it also relates amazing specific stories on philanthropy, crisis management and acts of kindness. As a current dean, I could not help but believe that this book was written specifically to help me. However, I can easily see how leaders and aspiring leaders in academic medicine and beyond would benefit from these insights.

David Allen Brenner, MD
Vice Chancellor for Health Sciences
Dean of the School of Medicine
at the University of California, San Diego

Written by one of this generations most successful academic leaders, this personal account extracts a host of useful principles of leadership from the first-hand ordeals he faced over many years of guiding a complex academic medical center through a myriad of foreseen and unforeseen challenges.

Jordan J. Cohen, MD
Professor of Medicine and Public Health
George Washington University
President Emeritus
Association of American Medical Colleges

Dr. Levey and his team elevated UCLA to the 3rd Best Medical Center in America. His book is a "must-read" for aspiring leaders in every walk of life — from business to government. Dr. Levey set high ethical standards and always had time for everyone in his organization. His goal was to help others achieve their dreams.

Gray Davis
37th Governor of the State of California

In my corporate and consulting experiences, I have been exposed to most of the significant books on leadership of the past two decades, and there have been a lot of them. Finally, we have Dr. Levey's personal memoir of how theory meets action within the complexity of a world class Academic Health Center.

Becoming the successful architect of synchrony (to borrow Levey's term) between the medical school and UCLA's major hospital was due to intentional leadership. *Never Be Afraid to Do the Right Thing* provides an essential guide for boards, CEOs, deans and aspiring leaders, and it is written with humility, honesty and a sense of humor which allows its lessons to be applied with that much more facility. A book that should be in everyone's library.

William M. Dwyer, MBA
President
Dwyer HC Strategist, LLC

Dr. Gerald Levey is one of America's great leaders. In *Never Be Afraid to Do the Right Thing*, you will learn how to take your leadership to the next level. Some of us were blessed to receive direct mentoring from Dr. Levey. For those who were not as fortunate, this book provides those jewels.

David T. Feinberg, MD, MBA
CEO, UCLA Hospital System

Dr. Levey has written an insightful and entertaining book on leadership, and it is a must-read for all those who aspire to leadership of large organizations.

David Geffen

Never Be Afraid to Do the Right Thing offers a lifetime's worth of experience from one of the most highly respected leaders in academic medicine. Dr. Gerald Levey's wisdom, humor and compassion shine through on every page as he presents clear, practical strategies for building an effective team, maintaining an institution's vision and handling tough decisions. There is no substitute for personal values in a leader and Dr. Levey's standards are of the highest order in ethics, integrity and work ethic. Academic medicine and the institutions where he has worked are fortunate to have had such an exemplary and visionary leader.

Antonio M. Gotto, Jr., MD, DPhil
Stephen and Suzanne Weiss Dean and Professor of Medicine
Weill Cornell Medical College
New York, NY

Dr. Levey has written an intensely personal account of his rise to the very pinnacle of American academic medicine. His humanism and values come through on every page and provide a compelling guide to established and aspiring leaders alike. While describing his own journey, Dr. Levey provides both a structured framework for leadership development and practical tips on how to manage the numerous challenges and opportunities that inevitably accompany such a journey. As a 'new' dean, I found the book inspirational and highly instructive.

Sam Hawgood, MBBS
Dean, University of California,
San Francisco School of Medicine
Vice Chancellor Medical Affairs,
University of California, San Francisco

As president and CEO of The Walt Disney Company, I have been fortunate to observe Dr. Levey's visionary leadership of UCLA's Academic Health Center for approximately the last ten years. *Never Be Afraid to Do the Right Thing* is an accurate reflection of his operating style and the principles he believes in. The book should be required reading for all those individuals in business, government and medicine who aspire to leadership.

The decision that Dr. Levey made to present his views of leadership against the backdrop of his personal history is particularly fascinating and I believe a masterful stroke for the importance and readability of the book. Without question, leaders such as Dr. Levey are crafted by life's events and others who impact their lives, such as role models and mentors. This book, I believe, will be very influential to the readers who are in the early stages of their careers in whatever their profession.

Robert A. Iger
President and CEO
The Walt Disney Company

The chapter devoted to fund-raising is instructive and perhaps unique in its approach. Dr. Levey was faced with an imperative to raise private donations to achieve an ambitious and game changing rebuilding of UCLA's Academic Health Center and he tells how he did it! This chapter by itself is worth the price of the book. A must read for all board of directors, leaders or aspiring leaders in every public and private institution.

I found Dr. Levey's discussion of his formative years a fascinating story. He brings to the forefront the things that occurred during his lifetime that in retrospect were transformative for his career and future success as a leader.

Dr. Levey's writing style is refreshing; the reader feels a special kinship with Dr. Levey and he makes you feel as if you are having a conversation with him.

Kirk Kerkorian
Chairman, President & CEO
Tracinda Corporation

Over the past fifteen years, I have had the great pleasure of working with Jerry Levey in my role as chair of the University of California Regents Health Services Committee and as a cancer patient advocate for the California Institute for Regenerative Medicine. Jerry is not only one of the finest individuals I have ever known, personally or professionally, he is also a brilliant doctor and an extraordinary leader. I was honored when he asked me to read the final draft of *Never Be Afraid to Do the Right Thing*. It was no surprise that the book turned out to be as insightful, informative and entertaining as its author.

Jerry's vision, intellect, integrity, experience, kindness and humor shine through on every page. This is a must-read for everyone. No matter what business you are in, you will be thoroughly enlightened by this personal memoir and management guide. I was particularly impressed with Jerry's insights into decision making, governance boards and the principles of fund-raising.

I know that you will enjoy reading *Never Be Afraid to Do the Right Thing* as much as I did — and I sincerely hope that this will be the first of many books from Dr. Levey.

Sherry Lansing
Former Chairman and CEO
Paramount Pictures
Founder of the Sherry Lansing Foundation

Dr. Levey's book has been a joy to read. It is an exceptionally valuable treatise on successful leadership of a flagship Academic Health Center. Its usefulness is universal to all complex organizations, and the style in which he has written his "how-to book" is a helpful guide for the conduct of a leadership role in any endeavor.

Healthcare today is undergoing a sea change. The requirements of superior leadership in the academic healthcare setting in the future are increasingly volatile and demanding, and present many challenges never before seen by today's leaders. Dr. Levey has been painstaking in documenting the principles, values, preparation and processes that have characterized his extensive experience. In doing so, he has provided a revealing history of the character of this great institution and of the leadership required to make it great.

Vernon R. Loucks, Jr.
Former Chairman & CEO
Baxter International, Inc.

Dr. Levey continues his great contributions to medicine, management and leadership by sharing his successful experience in this marvelous book.

In all knowledge-based disciplines, it seems that the least studied skill is the ability to lead the discipline for maximizing effect and benefit. Knowledge is the lead ingredient in progress, but leadership to synthesize and apply it is the ultimate value.

For so many important endeavors, be they economic, science, or medicine, the ability to apply the knowledge in order to create value and make improvements on behalf of our society is very important.

Many years ago, I had the privilege of studying under the famous management thought leader, Peter Drucker. Drucker often used the analogy of the orchestra leader to describe the importance of leadership to bring together people and knowledge in order to accomplish great things. Each musician has great knowledge of music and the instrument but, the orchestra leader brings the musicians and instruments together to produce a symphony.

Dr. Levey's life in medicine and leadership has been a journey of learning, successes and continuous improvement. The wealth of knowledge he has gained from the experience is an extremely valuable resource to those who wish to learn and improve their own abilities. Dr. Levey's generous sharing of his life experience and the success he has achieved is just another attribute of a tremendous leader.

While the content of Dr. Levey's book is medicine in the hospital and university setting, his insights on leadership and governance have a much broader application.

Many of his descriptions of effective leadership can be applied in business, government and other institutions as well.

The book reads as both a primer and a practical guide to the leadership skills required to be successful. Students of management and leadership will find real and interesting lessons even if they are not in medical or academic settings. Leadership skills have a universality that transcends the bounds of one's own discipline.

Another major dimension to effective leadership is ethical values and behavior. We too often see today in our institutions — business, government, academia — ethical lapses that test the credibility of those institutions.

Dr. Levey's own reputation for ethical leadership and his many insights into doing the right thing for the right reasons are powerful reminders for our own behavior.

The transfer of some of the tremendous wisdom he has accumulated over his long career to the reader is a gift that lasts a lifetime.

I have had the privilege of working with Dr. Levey in a business setting for many years. I have benefited from watching his thoughtful analysis of challenges, his attention to detail and his inquisitive nature. All of these attributes are wrapped in ethical and positive leadership. It has been an enjoyable learning experience.

The medical profession, as with many other professions, needs more knowledgeable sources for leadership. Dr. Levey's book certainly qualifies to be one of these sources.

One cannot say enough about the value of learning from success. I certainly recommend this book to anyone wanting to improve their leadership ability as well as gaining practical knowledge, based on real experience that can be immediately applied.

Thomas V. McKernan
CEO of AAA
Southern California

Jerry Levey's legendary leadership talents, passion for improving people's lives and humanity shine through in this book. Filled with wise observations, useful management guidance and even jokes, this is a book that provides invaluable insights on how to lead complicated organizations by tenaciously pursuing a vision, inspiring supporters, navigating excruciating choices and managing painful crises. There are leadership lessons here that apply to business and not-for-profit organizations, just as much as they do to complex healthcare systems.

Judy Olian
Dean and John E. Anderson Chair
UCLA Anderson School of Management

Dr. Gerald Levey is acknowledged as one of the outstanding Academic Health Center leaders of the modern era. Under his deft leadership, this great Center became measurably stronger and was "ahead of the curve" in anticipating the need for significant changes.

In *Never Be Afraid to Do the Right Thing*, Dr. Gerald Levey has written a remarkably comprehensive, detailed description of the principles and practices of effective leadership — as applied to UCLA's Academic Health Center. In my view, it is a "must-read" for all participants in the unique cultures of these centers — and in particular for actual and aspiring leaders. The narrative is replete with examples of challenging situations in which effective leadership was the limiting factor in achieving the desired outcomes. Adding to the book's appeal is its personal touch; a history of the key features of Dr. Levey's background and academic career which prepared him for AHC leadership and specific recognition of the many people who contributed so much to his personal development and to the success of the health center. The importance of Levey's message cannot be underestimated — it is particularly timely in light of current efforts to reform American healthcare. The fact is that the excellence of academic health centers is an absolute requirement for the future enhancement of health and healthcare.

William A. Peck, MD
Director, Center for Health Policy
Alan A. and Edith L. Wolff Distinguished
Professor of Medicine
Dean Emeritus, School of Medicine
Washington University, St. Louis, Missouri

Drawing from his transformative contributions to academic medicine, Dr. Levey has created a powerful and inspiring book of wisdom about leadership. An intriguing glimpse into what is required for success in a leading university health system, this book has lessons for those aspiring to lead, and those already in leadership roles, in any field. Dr. Levey documents his development as an esteemed dean and the insights that propelled his success. He generously shares his advice on how to "do the right thing." This should be required reading for anyone wanting to be a medical school dean and anyone trying to understand their medical school dean! The chapter on philanthropy is a must-read from one of the most successful fund-raisers of this era. Full of "pearls of wisdom," this book is fun to read and full of high-impact, practical advice — you will find yourself remembering Dr. Levey's advice frequently.

Claire Pomeroy, MD, MBA
Chief Executive Officer, UC Davis Health System
Vice Chancellor, Human Health Sciences
Dean, School of Medicine
University of California, Davis

No one has had a closer seat over the past two decades at advancing leading-edge healthcare than Dr. Gerald Levey, and this timely book provides readers with "floor seats" to his leadership insights. Learn how a great leader successfully blended vision, perseverance, teamwork, humility and humor to make lasting impacts in the world of healthcare and on the many people he touched.

Amir Dan Rubin
President and CEO
Stanford Hospital & Clinics

Dr. Levey's book well serves both theory and practice by covering a wide range of important issues for leaders of academic health centers. It is full of accumulated wisdom and, importantly, is based on Dr. Levey's strong conviction that the academic and clinical sides of the academic health center must be aligned to achieve true excellence. I recommend this book to those who aspire to leadership positions in academic medicine.

Steven A. Wartman, MD, PhD, MACP
President and CEO
Association of Academic Health Centers

ABOUT THE BOOK

In this business memoir, Dr. Levey shares with the reader lessons learned from many years of experience.

A trained internist and endocrinologist, an investigator at the Howard Hughes Medical Institute while at the University of Miami, a senior vice president for one of the world's leading pharmaceutical companies, chairman of the department of medicine at the University of Pittsburgh School of Medicine, Dr. Levey culminated his career as vice chancellor, Medical Sciences and dean of the David Geffen School of Medicine at UCLA.

During his long and illustrious career at UCLA, he re-built one of the world's premier academic health centers after the devastating Northridge earthquake in 1994.

The book is titled after Dr. Levey's favorite business admonishment, *Never Be Afraid to Do the Right Thing.* Healthcare executives should adopt the lessons in this book to take their leadership to the next level. While each chapter alone is worth the price of the book, as a former healthcare executive, I would encourage every healthcare leader to study the chapters entitled "Crisis Management" and "Fund-Raising."

The chapter on fund-raising expands ones vision on the potential of what can be done and hospital foundation leaders and board members would benefit from Dr. Levey's insight and direction. You can count on one hand the number of healthcare leaders that have had the tremendous successes in fund-raising that Dr. Levey has had.

Aspiring healthcare leaders should study this book as a primer on how to lead a healthcare organization, no matter how small or large, and remember: *Never Be Afraid to Do the Right Thing.*

Jerry F. Pogue
Publisher

FOREWORD

Who would have known?

I was surprised when I read the wonderful first draft of this book on leadership by Dr. Gerald S. Levey. I have known, worked for and worked with the man for over thirty years, first as head of the Division of Endocrinology and Metabolism when he was chairman of Internal Medicine at the University of Pittsburgh and then as executive associate dean at the David Geffen School of Medicine at UCLA (the position that he refers to throughout the book as his chief operating officer). During these years, I have watched Jerry work with the principles that he outlines in this book. And while at every step I marveled at his insight and analysis, he was so unassuming in his leadership that I put him among the "unconsciously competent." Yet, he has consciously put these principles down on paper and produced a treatise of guiding principles for those who aspire to be successful leaders in academic medicine.

He stayed true to principles he grew up with, "honesty is the best policy," "keep your word," and "don't make promises you can't keep." To these he added principles of his own that those of us who know him have incorporated as our own principles as well, "there is always time to think," "when in doubt go with your instincts" and the title of this book, "never be afraid to do the right thing," because "doing the right thing gives freedom of action and comfort at night."

The importance of applying these principles to the little things that occur every day, says Dr. Levey, is that these little things each day become the big things in life. Using these principles, even unfortunate, unpredictable and unwanted precipitating events have the potential to lead to wonderful outcomes. (An earthquake led to a new hospital.)

Don't be deceived and think that following these principles will make academic leadership easy. It is difficult; but, these principles can make academic leadership easier. One of the most important things a leader can do is build an efficient team. The team must be so well-known to and personally respected by the leader that no one doubts that every member of the team speaks for the leader. Recently I heard President Obama make the observation that the reason the presidency is a tough job is that only the difficult decisions end up on his desk. Similarly, Dr. Levey made the observation that a leader cannot be involved in most of the decisions that are made in an academic medical center. Most of the decisions will be made by members of the team. The leader must recognize that although each member of the team works together, they also individually have dreams and aspirations of their own. Over time an emotional bond develops between the leader and the team members and the leader can encourage their dreams and promote their aspirations, even if it means some members move on.

Certainly every era has its sense of change, but the present era seems especially dynamic with a new health care delivery system, advances in genetic medicine and the emergence of stem cell research. Dr. Levey points out that academic medical centers must remain steadfastly committed to the fundamental truths — research creates knowledge, education disseminates knowledge, patient care applies knowledge and public service utilizes all three. The next generation of leaders must understand the institution they are joining even before they arrive. They must see the institution as an important part of the academic and civic community. Resources will be limited, so collaborative work with other schools and colleges in their institution and with other academic medical centers nationally and internationally is necessary for success. This new generation of leaders will face unprecedented challenges and must be rigorously screened for the skill sets and traits delineated here in this book and that are needed to succeed. These skill sets may be honed in any of a variety of positions and experiences other than in academic medicine. Those assuming leadership positions in academic medicine must have a long-term view because as Dr. Levey points out, the times are too perilous to have leaders with only a short tenure.

An essential part of the leader being a member of the civic community is developing a base of philanthropic supporters who will understand that the goals of the academic medical center are consistent with their goals for the community. The donor chapter is one of the great chapters of this book. I won't repeat here Dr. Levey's eight principles for fund-raising, but this chapter should be required reading for every leader of an academic medical center and every member of the development staff that supports them.

I close with a few personal notes. It helps one to develop into the personal leader that Dr. Levey has become if you grew up like he did in the era when your family physician was a respected "member of your family" and a pillar of the community. And, discrimination that he felt as a Jew and observed in opinions of others about Catholics, women, and African-Americans may make someone a kinder person; one who quotes easily Yogi Berra and Stephen Covey; one who has a sense of humor and can tell the appropriate joke in proper context at the appropriate time and place. (Incidentally, if you can read his one-liners in the chapter on humor without laughing out loud, you need to develop some relaxation exercises.)

I return to the opinion I had throughout the years that Dr. Levey was "unconsciously competent." Indeed, when Jerry first told me, "never be afraid to do the right thing," I thought it was a spontaneous personal insight that he shared only with me. I was somewhat jealous when I learned that other people were also given this verbal gem. But I was not completely off base in the "unconsciously competent" opinion. Dr. Levey notes that the first time he really recognized the extent to which he had passed his personal value system onto others was in the comments of colleagues when he was being honored as he stepped down from his position as vice chancellor and dean. So, he decided to "sharpen my thinking on what happened during the fifteen years at UCLA" and write about it. In doing so, he has produced a book for anyone aspiring to a role as a leader; to help them recognize traits that will make them successful. He reminds us, "an incredible amount of work ethic is required, the time demands are phenomenal, the evenings on the dinner circuit are beyond expectations," but "If you're prepared, experienced and motivated, chances are good for success."

I have lifted freely and unabashedly from Dr. Levey's text (with permission). To get the whole story in context, read on with pleasure.

Alan G. Robinson, MD
Associate Vice Chancellor, Medical Sciences
Executive Associate Dean,
UCLA School of Medicine

PREFACE

I recently completed my three term, fifteen year tenure as the vice chancellor for Medical Sciences and dean of the David Geffen School of Medicine. About half-way through my last term, I informed the UCLA Chancellor, Dr. Gene Block, of my intent to step down from my administrative position. I thought that after such a long tenure the time was right; the many challenges that were facing me in 1994 beginning with the aftermath of the Northridge Earthquake had been largely overcome or would be with the completion of the new earthquake resistant (must withstand at least earthquake magnitude 8 on the Richter Scale) Ronald Reagan UCLA Medical Center which would be completed in June 2008.

As I thought about retirement from my position, I spent many hours reflecting on my life after administration and I came to the conclusion that if I wanted to continue to have a useful professional life and to remain intellectually stimulated, I needed to undertake projects that I had never done before. Therefore I decided on two challenging projects focused on leadership. The first project was to write a book and the second was to design a course for medical students and possibly for students in the UCLA College and/or the Anderson School of Management at UCLA. I felt that the book needed to come first because it would ultimately be the underpinning for any course or courses that I developed and I needed to sharpen my thinking on what happened during my fifteen years at UCLA, why and how it happened, and where and how I developed the personal qualities necessary for successfully leading a large and complicated organization.

In writing this book, I was also confronted with other challenges. The first was writing a book in which I put forth the conclusions about my success and yet did not make me appear egotistical or as if I was writing an infomercial for UCLA and its medical sciences. The second was making it clear to those who aspire to leadership of any organization, especially one so large and complex like an academic health center, and to all the readers of this book, the critical role played by the team that is put in place by the leader and the necessity for the individual members of the team to share your vision for the organization and your personal values discussed in detail in Chapter Three such as honesty, integrity, work ethic, truthfulness and commitment to excellence. In effect, being a successful leader is like being the conductor of a symphony. Day in and day out how the team performs both as a group and as individuals is what determines the success of the organization and achieving the goals and vision set by the leader. The leader's team members deserve and need your respect, mentoring, approval, recognition of their achievements and also your patience and guidance when they perhaps miss the mark. They need to create their own micro-environment to grow and develop and achieve their career aspirations. I was blessed to have the team I was able to construct at UCLA. I will always be in their debt for their successes, hard work and loyalty and respect for me and the institution. In the School of Medicine, I believe I had the finest executive associate dean and group of senior associate, associate and assistant deans and extraordinary basic science and clinical chairs who were truly "world-class." The chief executive officer of our hospital system was exceptional and his hospital team served with distinction. My entire team in the School of Medicine and hospital system will always have my respect, love, admiration and heartfelt thanks.

The third challenge was having to make the decision early on to write the core of this book as an autobiography. Therefore the book is not an academic exercise but in essence it is a "how-to book" lived and visualized through one person who successfully accomplished leadership of a highly complex academic health center. I believe deeply that my formative years and my family history had much to do with my ultimate accomplishments in life. I owe more than I can adequately portray or repay to my parents, the late Gertrude and Jacob Levey, and to my wife of fifty years, Dr. Barbara Levey. I also was blessed with an array of mentors in my professional life that extended from medical school to the present. All of these people gave a part of their lives to me in an attempt to enable me to reach my full potential. Writing about them and recalling them in my mind has produced conflicting emotions of gratitude, respect and love, and yet a profound sadness because most of them are now deceased and many of them could not be witness to my successes. This sadness is most profound with regard to my parents, especially my father, who died when I was a teenager. Therefore I recognize that this book had to be in part a testimonial to my parents, my wife and my professors because without them my life would have been far different.

I also knew the book would be a challenge from at least one other aspect. Since I am a physician with broad experience in medicine, administration and dealing with people from all strata and walks of life, it would be imperative to have some chapters relate not just to my "professional club" of medical administrators, but also to the general business community and layman who are interested in leadership qualities regardless of the organization. In other words, the book must successfully cover the broad map of how to succeed as a leader and to have a theme of leadership bind the chapters together for every reader and their own specific area of interest, even though it is primarily about leadership of a large academic health center. For a novice writer such as myself, it has been a challenge and I hope you, the readers, find the reading easy, interesting and above all informative.

Finally, the preface would not be complete without a clear delineation of what I want to achieve by writing this book. The following are my goals and in reading the preface, I hope the goals I articulate serve to stimulate you even further to read this book.

GOALS

First and foremost, I want the reader to recognize the many traits that any given individual must possess to be a successful leader. I hope recognition of these traits translates to a greater understanding of what it takes to be a successful leader not only in medicine but whatever organization with which you are involved or working in, at whatever level. I hope the book will make the reader reflect on people you admire in medicine, business, politics, a charitable organization, restaurant, etc. I am certain you will recognize the core traits even though a leader in medicine may well display certain specific qualities inherent in running a large medical organization.

Although writing a broadly applicable book on leadership is a worthy goal, I want to make clear to the reader that my second goal is to help define the generation of leaders and leadership for medical organizations like academic health centers. Hospitals and hospital systems are complicated and the seamless incorporation and integration of them within the academic components of an academic health center is essential and challenging. The medical school and its affiliated hospital or hospital system share the common goals of training the next generation of physicians and scientists, to foster pioneering research to ultimately provide treatments and cures for disease and to excel in the delivery of the finest patient care. On the other hand, the financial issues that are of concern to hospitals can trigger conflicts that may result in tensions between a school and hospital especially regarding the appropriate support dedicated to the medical school by the hospital. It is a formidable task to serve as a leader of this type of organization and a major effort is required to keep the various components of the academic health center headed in the right direction in order successfully achieve all of the goals.

Third, I want this book to serve as a portrait for recognizing those who have the most potential for leadership. I hope the book will lead to courses to help train the present and future generation of leaders, to help universities and other organizations, their search committees and search firms that aid them in their selection process, to identify individuals to lead their organization who possess the right traits to maximize their potential to lead and succeed.

Fourth, it is my hope and intent to convince you that leadership is ultimately all about caring for the people in your organization. What matters is that each individual leader's value system includes honesty, integrity, ethical and moral values, respect for all employees and, at the same time, a sense of humor that humanizes the leader. These values are indispensible to the support system to enable the leader to construct a vision and mission statement for an organization and to enable that organization to have a successful product generation, whether the product be new physicians and scientists, new therapies that cure disease or whatever specific product the business produces.

Fifth, this book is written for physicians, healthcare executives, board members of healthcare organizations, healthcare department managers, healthcare foundation leaders, foundation trustees, nurses, medical students, allied healthcare members and anyone interested in the principles of leadership in business or government.

I hope you, as a reader of this book, will find this preface helpful in understanding its contents. I also hope you enjoy reading the book as much as I enjoyed writing it.

DEDICATION

This book is dedicated to my wife of fifty years, Dr. Barbara Levey. The constants in my life have been her unflagging support and love, her sense of humor and wisdom.

ACKNOWLEDGEMENTS

I want to acknowledge the extraordinary efforts of my assistant, Joanne Loupee, who typed and retyped this manuscript and put up with this novice author as he worked on his first book. Her moral support and confidence that the book would be successful were greatly appreciated.

Four individuals were reviewers and read the entire text including Drs. Alan Robinson, Stanley Korenman, Peter Whybrow and Irwin Klein; their comments made this a better book. I also want to acknowledge the input of Dr. Barbara Levey, Judith Rothman, Joyce Fried, Dr. Gary Small, Judith Consales and Nancy Sacks who provided important input for specific chapters.

A special thanks to Dr. Pauline Chen who was extraordinarily helpful in getting me started on the road to becoming a published author.

I would also like to give a special thank you to two of my colleagues, Dale Tate and Dr. Thomas Rosenthal, who wrote and shared their exceptional expertise in Chapter Thirteen, "Crisis Management."

CHAPTER ONE

THE SHAPING OF A FUTURE LEADER

In deciding to write a book on leadership, I wanted the book to be autobiographical. I've never taken a course in leadership, and as far as I know, during my tenure there weren't any. I learned on the job. As I reflected on my career and my years of service as a leader, it was evident to me that "I am what I am" was dictated by forces both internal and external to my environment. These forces in effect shaped me for my future professional life and that is why I start this chapter at the beginning of my life.

Lessons from My Early Life

I was born on January 9, 1937. My debut into the world, the day my sister was scheduled to celebrate her fifth birthday, was less than a hit. I unintentionally rained on her parade, forcing the cancellation of her birthday party. Despite this and happily, my sister and I remain close and (almost) never forget each other's birthdays.

I knew I wanted to become a physician when I was four years old. My reason was our family physician, Dr. Samuel Rosenstein, a pediatrician who had cared for my father and his siblings when they emigrated from Russia and for all their children, including my sister and me. Our physician until we reached the age of 21, Dr. Rosenstein practiced medicine until he was 92 years old! He was an amazing man of whom I was totally in awe. In my mind, he was the human personification of God. Although he had an office, Dr. Rosenstein was recognized not only for his compassion, intelligence, and professionalism, but for his house calls. He performed a number of medical and surgical procedures on me on the kitchen table, literally. He set my broken nose when I was six or seven-years-old. When I almost severed my finger in a car door, he sewed what remained of it back in place on the kitchen table. And when I broke my collarbone climbing around in a lumberyard, he set the fracture on the same kitchen table. I also remember quite vividly the various times my mom asked him to make a house call because I had a high fever.

Dr. Rosenstein was wise and dedicated and I think what amazed me even more than his spectacular bedside manner and calm and reassuring demeanor was that he kept up with the science of the day. When he decided against using antibiotics for one of my illnesses, I remember him telling my mom that he didn't want to abuse these new drugs, tetracycline and penicillin, because he had read in the medical literature that the bacteria have a way of becoming resistant to them. This man was my role model and I knew that I wanted to follow in his footsteps. I don't remember ever wanting to be anything else in my life but a physician.

In grammar school, I skipped from kindergarten to second grade and when I graduated from grammar school I was voted "most likely to succeed." That was a good start! In high school, I was sports editor of the school newspaper and in that role I reported to people in management, a useful skill, since I would end up spending my entire career reporting to management, until I became management.

Following high school graduation, I began my undergraduate studies at Cornell University. Midway through my first year, I almost flunked out. Coming from an inner city high school, it took me almost a full year to get the knack of studying under pressure and competing with the best students from all over the country. I told my parents after four months at Cornell that I was on academic probation. Both my parents were totally supportive of me. Years later my mother told me that she had been really upset but my father had said at the time, "don't worry about the boy, he will be fine." Thank God for giving me my dad and mom; they really saved my life.

When I was eighteen-years-old and finishing my second year at Cornell, my father died. We were not wealthy; my dad had graduated Rutgers Newark night school and had become a lawyer with expertise in constitutional law. He was the only child sent to college by his family because he was the youngest. He was a remarkable man who understood me, my age, my fallibilities and my potential. His death almost stopped my career in its tracks by its suddenness and financial implications.

From that point on, my mom, who had only a high school diploma and never worked outside the home, dedicated her life to financing my education. She was insistent that I start my working life unburdened by this expense. Although the costs were vastly less in those days than they are now, it was not easy for her to put the financing together. But she did, getting a job at Dickinson High School as an administrative secretary, and because of her support, I was able to complete my education without debt.

The next phase of my life and another bump in the road occurred when I applied to medical school and encountered prejudices that I never expected. First, I found that many of the surrounding states did not want additional students from New Jersey to enter their medical schools. I was told by several schools at which I interviewed that the general feeling was that New Jersey should start a medical school and take care of its own students. I was also told there were fairly tightly restricted quotas on how many Jewish students were accepted.

Fortunately, I was accepted at a new school, the Seton Hall College of Medicine in Jersey City, a member of the second class admitted. The school was sponsored by the Archdiocese of northern New Jersey and was a major strategic initiative of Archbishop McNulty of New Jersey, who started the medical school to enable Catholics, Jews, African Americans and women, the discriminated groups during my era, to study medicine. When I was admitted, I was determined I wasn't going to screw this up. I finished second in my class, a far cry from my record at Cornell.

At Seton Hall I was essentially adopted by the faculty because I was a student who they viewed as having high potential for a career in academic medicine. There were at least five senior faculty who cared enough about me to spend hours ensuring my future success by showing me the keys to developing a successful career in academic medicine.

Dr. Harold Jeghers, the chief of medicine, took me with him on many consultations to hospitals in the New Jersey and New York area and I had the opportunity to witness his clinical brilliance at the bedside. Dr. John Calabro helped me and taught me to write a clinical manuscript and I was fortunate to have two publications co-authored with him by the time I was a first year resident. Dr. Richard Chambers guided me through a field study of an outbreak of Eastern Equine Encephalitis and was always patient and understanding as I learned on the job how to do a clinical study. This study led to a co-authored presentation to the American Neurological Association in my senior year. Dr. Carroll Leevey was my role model for excellence in teaching rounds and over the years successfully nominated me for every important society in internal medicine. For years after I had left Seton Hall, and in many ways, he was like a surrogate father.

Part of my determination to succeed came from the love of my life, Dr. Barbara Levey, whom I met in my senior year at Cornell. Barbara, an outstanding student, was a real pioneer. She went to SUNY (State University of New York) Upstate Medical School in Syracuse, and was the only woman graduate in her medical school class of 120. She was an inspiration to me then and has continued to remain so; someone who has always done her best to see that I achieved all of my goals in life, including our geographic odyssey that neither of us could have predicted. She was able to overcome prejudices directed at women and reached the pinnacle in her specialty of clinical pharmacology.

Evolution of my Career Goals

During my internship at Jersey City Medical Center, Dr. Philip Henneman, the chief of endocrinology advised me that if I was serious about wanting a career in academic medicine, I had to learn how to do research and become a physician scientist. He recommended that I apply to Harvard Medical School for postdoctoral training. After my internship, I applied and was accepted to the biological chemistry department at Harvard Medical School where I spent two years as a postdoctoral fellow learning the tools of a basic scientist. I then completed my residency training at Massachusetts General Hospital. Following this, I went to the National Institutes of Health in Bethesda as a lieutenant commander in the United States Public Health Service where I spent four years. It was there that I further refined my research skills but also saw patients and had an excellent clinical experience in endocrinology.

At the age of thirty-three, I accepted an offer from the University of Miami School of Medicine to join their faculty as an associate professor of medicine. In addition, I was nominated for and received a competitive Howard Hughes Medical Investigatorship. Nine years later, in 1979, I was a candidate for the University of Miami chair of medicine. Additionally, I had been offered a chairmanship at the University of Pittsburgh; my preference was to stay at the University of Miami, however, life is unpredictable. I wasn't selected as the chair of medicine and I accepted the offer from the University of Pittsburgh, which presented an opportunity to rebuild a distinguished Department of Medicine. The thought of leaving Miami for a cold climate was not big on the hit parade for me or my family, but Barbara and the children were willing to move so I could, as my son put it, "have my shot."

The University of Pittsburgh gave me the opportunity to develop my administrative and leadership skills. As chairman of the Department of Medicine, I was expected to rebuild and energize a once great department and restore its quality and sense of purposeful direction to achieve academic excellence. I had to recruit a number of new division chiefs and restructure the department along a theme of general internal medicine serving as the core. I also had the opportunity to initiate a clinical investigator training program and to be the director of a second year multi-departmental course for the medical students. The University gave me the opportunity to do some fund-raising and to realize the necessity of developing the programs that you wish to develop more completely. I learned to manage a large budget, to eliminate an inherited departmental deficit, and I gained the invaluable experience of forming a practice plan.

In my thirteenth year at Pitt, I was contacted by the pharmaceutical giant, Merck, and offered the position of senior vice president for Medical and Scientific Affairs. My time at Merck was a fabulous experience where I learned to run a major organization by observing how the company was led by its CEO, Dr. Roy Vagelos.

In December of 1993, I received a call from the head of the search committee at UCLA asking me to interview for the job of dean of the

School of Medicine and provost for Medical Sciences. I was captivated by the opportunities presented by this job because I had begun to dream about running a major academic medical center. This job was perfect because it included not only responsibility for the medical school, but also oversight of the practice plans and the hospital system. And, as they say, the rest is history.

As I think about my early life through graduation from Cornell, there are several life experiences that were pivotal in helping me prepare for my ultimate job as leader of an academic medical center.

The first was that I wanted a career in medicine and felt passionate about becoming a physician. I locked in on that goal and never wavered in achieving it. Clearly I benefitted by experiencing firsthand the need for and importance of a role model. Our family physician fulfilled that role although he was probably not aware of his impact on my life. Dr. Rosenstein possessed the essence of a high-quality practitioner: excellent communication with the patient and his/her family, a professional but caring bedside manner and a superior knowledge base of medicine. He was wise in the application of new knowledge as evidenced by his reluctance to use new antibiotics indiscriminately.

The second was experiencing the shock of losing my father suddenly. His unexpected death had a negative impact on me as a child. While learning to cope with adversity precipitated by his death, I also experienced the love of my mom who turned to full-time employment to enable my educational goals to be met. Ultimately, I had to focus more intently on my goals to complete my education successfully and become a physician. Passion for my chosen profession, persistence when faced with adversity and the need to overcome it, the importance of a role model, and the love and support of my parents and spouse were critical lessons that I learned beginning at a young age.

The third was the experiences as a postdoctoral fellow in Biological Chemistry at Harvard coupled with four additional years at the National Institute of Health establishing me as a physician-scientist in the area of cyclic nucleotides and hormone action. This laid a firm foundation for my understanding of the power of science as it pertains to clinical medicine. I understood what was required to establish a first-class research enterprise including research facilities, advanced technology, and the necessity for interdisciplinary research. Today I realize this is critical information for someone with the responsibility of running a large academic medical center.

The fourth was experiencing the challenges and successes of rebuilding an organization, in my case, the Department of Medicine at the University of Pittsburgh School of Medicine. I also was involved with, and observed the massive reorganization and development of the entire academic health center at the University of Pittsburgh by the late Dr. Thomas Detre and Mr. Jeffrey Romoff, including a total makeover of the hospitals, the medical school, and the practice plans. It was Dr. Detre who had recruited me to the University of Pittsburgh when I was at the University of Miami. He was indefatigable and brilliant, and had a laser vision for the goals of the University of Pittsburgh School of Medicine and Hospital System. He could énvision the future and he was determined to change the culture of the University of Pittsburgh to the modern, dynamic institution it has become. It was a very special learning experience for me.

Thomas Detre was my friend and mentor. One day in 1989, we had one of these "what do I want to be when I grow up" chats. I told him ultimately I wanted to run an academic medical center just like him. He said in his Hungarian accent, that it was unlikely that I would get such a job with only the experience of running a moderate size Department of Medicine. His frankness took me by surprise and I asked him how one acquires the right experiences. I told him I had visited about a dozen schools looking at deanship positions and didn't want to leave for those jobs because most deans appeared to be unhappy. The conversation with Dr. Detre didn't go any further at that time, but two years later I received a career-changing call from Dr. R. Gordon Douglas. Dr. Douglas was a former chair of medicine at Cornell Medical College. When he called me, he was the senior vice president for Medical and Scientific Affairs at Merck & Company, soon to be appointed president of Merck's vaccine division. He asked if I would be interested in interviewing for the job of senior vice president for Medical and Scientific Affairs. I accepted, seeing this as an opportunity for "that extra something" Dr. Detre had described, that would put me in a better position to be selected to run a very large enterprise.

The scope of my job at Merck was international, involving world-wide clinical trials and participation on strategic committees of the Merck research laboratories. I considered myself fortunate to be there when the company's CEO was Dr. Roy Vagelos, who not only headed one of America's great companies, but was the most successful CEO in the pharmaceutical industry between 1984 and 1994. He had incredible vision about the current situation and what it needed to become; he worked hard, was unflappable under stress and was a master of communications. The various meetings at Merck, including management council meetings, were models of civility and decorum. The productive discussions were something I had not seen in the various academic environments in which I had previously participated. Everyone, from the office staff to the CEO, knew where we were going at Merck and why the enterprise must be one for all and all for one. It was an exciting place to be and, in actuality, my three years there were, in effect, a sabbatical. What I didn't know at the time was that the "sabbatical" was about to end. In retrospect, Drs. Detre and Vagelos were the last chapter of my tutorial on how to be the leader of a large organization. They set the stage for me to complete, with one more stop, my geographic odyssey. That stop would be Los Angeles.

CHAPTER TWO

ACADEMIC HEALTH CENTERS

Academic Health Centers (AHCs) arose in the early to mid-twentieth century and have become the core upon which much of the modern American healthcare system is built. This is an especially important chapter for the reader who is unfamiliar with the governance structure of medicine because this structure has been fundamental to the successes of the present healthcare system. The "Affordable Care Act," passed into law in 2010, will require a highly-trained, open-minded, creative core of leaders who will be expected to lead the medical profession to preserve what is good in this governance structure while at the same time achieving what will be required to productively and successfully adapt to the new challenges that will occur supplemental to the mandated changes of the Affordable Care Act. Medical practice will change and emphasize primary care and to a greater extent prevention; the composition of the workforce required will necessitate more generalists, nurses and physician assistants, and there will be adjustments in reimbursement policy to name only a few of the changes.

The greatest and most basic challenges I had as the leader of an academic health center were to ensure a harmonious, focused view of medical practice, research and education and to foster "one for all and all for one" camaraderie and understanding between the School of Medicine and its leaders and faculty and the hospital system leadership. It required my constant attention over the years and occasional changes in personnel. With this prologue, we can begin our discussion below that I hope will make clear this complex yet fragile structure that has served medicine and the country so well.

The basic and most simple definition of an AHC is an allopathic or osteopathic medical school and its primary teaching hospital or hospitals; this configuration is also referred to as an Academic Medical Center (AMC). Traditionally, AHCs are more complex than AMCs because they encompass one or more health profession schools such as Pharmacy, Dentistry, Public Health and Nursing. Nevertheless, the core component is the School of Medicine for both the AMC and AHC. AMCs/AHCs house the majority of the country's leadership pool of physicians and scientists, including the deans of the various schools, the hospital and health system CEOs, department chairs, faculty and those who aspire to leadership positions. For the purposes of clarity, I will refer to the institutions covered in this book as AHCs.

The AHCs have contributed in a very important way to advances in our healthcare system; they have produced a supply of well-trained physicians for the United States as good as any in the world. Working in concert with subspecialty boards and state medical licensing agencies, AHCs have adopted and supported rigorous standards for accreditation of schools of medicine as well as for licensing examinations, specialty board certification and recertification. Under the leadership of the AHCs, extraordinary growth of generalists and subspecialists has occurred as well as development of excellent continuing medical education programs.

Significantly, AHCs have also produced a steady supply of well-trained scientists and physician-scientists. More than half of the Nobel Prizes in medicine and physiology have been received by physician-scientists and scientists residing in the large AHCs. Researchers in AHCs have set ambitious goals to conduct research that is applicable to patients (translational research, "bench to bedside") with remarkable results. The research effort has been creative, entrepreneurial and bold, and has changed our understanding of human disease in relatively few decades. The emergence of the modern pharmaceutical industry with its emphasis on research leading to new drug development has produced an unprecedented partnership with AHCs and has become a remarkable success story by developing new therapies for patients. Many clinical trials conducted in the United States are led by or utilize AHC physicians. AHCs have played critical roles in local communities by providing services to the uninsured, underserved and for the less fortunate in society. They are powerful forces in both local and national economics and are often the largest employers in the many cities in which they are located.

Finally, the world-class, research-driven patient care delivered in AHCs by dedicated physicians, nurses and staff is renowned for its cutting edge diagnostic and therapeutic agents and for the procedures that have saved countless lives.

AHCs have become large complex businesses, and as such, they present the same internal tensions of a business. On occasion the academic and clinical missions do not work together ideally, thus negatively impacting the organization. The governance of these large and complex AHCs and the diverse and robust mission they represent demand their leadership provides excellence in management in a challenging environment. Some governance structures have worked properly, while some have not. Suboptimal governance generally leads to a lack of cohesion of the organization and failure to achieve the critical organizational goals.

The governance structure I worked under during the 15½ years I served as vice chancellor for Medical Sciences and dean of the David Geffen School of Medicine at UCLA was based on the early success of the models of the Pennsylvania State University College of Medicine, the University of Pennsylvania School of Medicine and Duke University School of Medicine in which one individual is given the oversight of the entire medical complex. In my case, I had oversight of UCLA's world-renowned Ronald Reagan UCLA Medical Center, Santa Monica UCLA Medical Center and Orthopaedic Hospital, Mattel Children's Hospital, and the Stewart and Lynda Resnick Neuropsychiatric Hospital as well as the Faculty Practice Group and the David Geffen School of Medicine at UCLA. I did not run the hospital system; it was directed by a CEO who reported directly to me. The crux of my responsibility was to ensure that the goals of the medical school and hospital were in synchrony and that resources were allocated to support programs and people appropriate for fulfilling UCLA's overall mission in the medical sciences.

The sizes of the budgets of the AHCs are largely dependent on their hospital(s), the size and quality of their research enterprises and the extent to which the many components of the AHCs are owned by the university. The budget for which I had responsibility exceeded $2.5 billion, making it the equivalent of at least a Fortune 500 company. Our leadership team had a special collegiality and chemistry, a plethora of financial skills, and a shared vision as to how and what to support with available resources, which provided proper direction to the organization and prevented dysfunction between the academic and business side of the AHC.

My concept of the mission of a 21st century AHC is shown in tabular form below.

The Mission of Academic Health Centers in the 21st century includes:

- Training physicians and scientists
- Performing cutting edge translational research
- Delivering the highest quality patient care
- Recruiting and retaining outstanding physicians and scientists
- Maintaining the highest ethical standards
- Promoting the health and welfare of the community
- Cultivating philanthropy
- Developing a diverse faculty and student body
- Educating the public regarding AHCs and their functions

The three core elements of the mission are in many ways the same as they have been has been for the last seventy years: training and educating the next generation of physicians, physician-scientists, and scientists; providing outstanding patient care; and maintaining a microenvironment that enables the biomedical research enterprise to thrive and produce state-of-the-art medical advances.

AHCs must adhere to a clearly stated commitment to maintain the highest ethical standards and to identify and eliminate conflicts of interest that periodically flare and cause consternation and concern by the general public and government agencies. Fulfilling this part of the mission requires transparency of the business side of academia, especially relationships between the AHC and the pharmaceutical, biotech and medical device industries.

At least 40 percent of the care provided to the underserved and uninsured individuals in our communities is provided by AHCs who are the major safety net providers. Many of our students and faculty members volunteer to help those less fortunate. This commitment is required to maintain public trust and support.

Developing other revenue streams such as philanthropy is critical to the AHC bottom line. The nature of what AHCs do in education, research and patient care provides a natural focus for goal-directed philanthropy. This endeavor requires commitment on the part of AHC leadership and faculty, including investment in the creation of a professional development office. Maximal effort to develop philanthropic support should yield enormous growth potential. I will discuss this in greater detail in a later chapter. One thing is certain — with declining support from federal and state sources, the need for philanthropy will become increasingly more apparent to all and will be of utmost importance for maintaining the infrastructure of AHCs and making them competitive on a global basis in terms of resources, quality of educational programs, and patient care delivered.

I quickly learned how important a role philanthropy would play in achieving success and realized it would occupy more of my time than I originally thought. The primary concern for me as leader was to be highly responsive to requests for medical help and to ensure that those in need, rich or poor, were directed to our physicians and medical services expeditiously; and secondly, that we were recognized by the surrounding community as being highly responsive and that we provided the finest care. I organized a division of special services that developed, in retrospect, into a concierge medical practice.

The diversity of our students and faculty is a national concern. America is a multicultural society and AHCs need to provide the general public with a representative ethnic and racial workforce of physicians and physician-scientists. Achieving diversity has proven to be a challenging area and a difficult task. It will take time, commitment and possibly a complete overhaul of the public education system in the United States to accomplish this. A clear statement to this effect as part of the AHC mission is therefore appropriate.

Considering the complexity of AHCs, it is important that the public and our local, state, and federal legislatures know what we do and why we do it. We must not be taken for granted because too much is at stake for the future of AHCs. It seems paradoxical that AHCs always seem to have both a bright future and equally ominous challenges ahead.

Healthcare reform is one of these paradoxical challenges. While many parts of the healthcare system need to be repaired, all the worthy elements in our healthcare system must be identified and nurtured. Some of the challenges as I see them are:

- Increasing the affordability and accessibility of health insurance.
- Achieving changes in Medicare and Medicaid that enhance efficiency and provide acceptable reimbursement to physicians and hospitals.
- Reimbursing medical advances that represent the future successes of translational research.
- Defining a more prominent role for preventive medicine given the principle that it is far less costly to prevent disease than to treat it. This will involve identifying approaches including, but not limited to, nutrition, smoking cessation, environmental pollution, vaccine development, and the emerging field of genetic medicine. The diagnostic and therapeutic tools provided by a genetic approach to disease prevention must be both available and affordable.
- Supporting medical education and developing a physician work force appropriate for the 21st century. Work force shortages exist not only in primary care but also in the subspecial-

ties. Miscalculations (either under or over) of the projected shortages must be avoided.

- Bringing medical services to underserved areas.

- Maintaining the fiscal integrity of NIH and ensuring its ability to sustain growth of biomedical research in order to fuel the generation of new knowledge that will lead to new cures and new diagnostic modalities.

- Assuring affordability and accessibility of new diagnostic and therapeutic interventions.

- Accommodating both the academic and business sides of medicine and industry by managing conflicts of interest.

- Keeping pharmaceutical companies viable through a period of great change and nurturing the partnership with academe that produces medications for our patients.

All of this will require a special excellence in leadership and development of leadership skills in individuals who wish to lead the AHCs and the healthcare industry now and into the future.

CHAPTER THREE

PRIMER FOR ASPIRING LEADERS

In 2003 I was invited by Dean Allen Lichter to serve as visiting dean at the University of Michigan School of Medicine. I readily accepted Dean Lichter's invitation. In preparing a formal lecture, I chose the title "One Dean's Perspective on the Medical Deanship." As I became involved in preparing my speech, it evolved into one of the most important lectures I have given in my career, representing the first steps in formalizing my thoughts about the constellation of character traits and qualities that translate to successful leadership within the challenging environment presented by an AHC. The first two or three decades of the 21st century are likely to be an exceptionally challenging period for American medicine due largely to a reformed healthcare delivery system, a plethora of advances from the scientific laboratories across the country, application of genetic medicine to everyday clinical practice and the emergence of stem cell research. Therefore the personal qualities and value systems that portend successful management of these large, multi-mission AHCs must be identified and, if possible, taught to those who aspire to lead and those who need to have their skills refined. Search committees, search firms and governing boards to which the AHCs report should be cognizant of these qualities when making hiring decisions regarding leaders of these organizations.

Within this chapter, the components of *Personal Qualities for Successful Leadership* are found in Table One and the *Principles for Effective Leadership* are depicted in Table Two. Before I discuss these various values and principles however, I want to provide a description of some of the challenges that occurred unexpectedly during my first year at UCLA that are illustrative of a sudden change in priorities and the need for adaptability on the part of the leader. My original job description was easily understood and relatively straightforward, however, UCLA's AHC underwent a transformational change precipitated by the 1994 Northridge Earthquake. During the time I interviewed for the position of vice chancellor for Medical Sciences and dean of the David Geffen School of Medicine (January 11, 1994 to May 1994), the verbal reports I received indicated that the impact of the Northridge earthquake was not disruptive on the future operations of the UCLA Medical Center which was considered usable and the cost of repairs manageable. However, as time went by and the structural engineering firms and the federal government probed deeper into the condition of the building, it became evident that shear wall strength had lessened significantly and by the mid-way point of my first year, it was becoming clear to everyone that the damage was far more extensive than originally anticipated. By the end of the year, it was considered likely that it would be too expensive and impractical to continue to conduct patient care operations while renovating the hospital. Patients and staff exposure to dust and noise, among other inconveniencies, would have been too dangerous. Although I wasn't thinking of my job duties at the time, the effect on my job description was such that it changed the job description the proverbial 180 degrees. I was required to morph into a major fund-raiser, involve myself in issues with FEMA and provide oversight to ensure that neither the hospital construction nor all the problems that would arise from constructing a new facility would negatively impact the campus. Our skilled Capital Programs team became indispensable colleagues and partners with their wealth of knowledge regarding earthquakes and building safety. The time commitments that were required over the next fourteen years, from site identification, architect selection, construction company selection and then the countless hours of planning and meetings once construction of the new hospital was underway, were enormous. Similar scenarios were also true for the research buildings that were simultaneously being planned and constructed. Time spent fund-raising was amazing in hours and intensity. Yet it was quite clear that accomplishing our mission was another opportunity of a lifetime because we would be able — with adequate funding from FEMA, donors and debt service — to construct a world-class hospital facility; a new facility that would be, for all intents and purposes, as earthquake proof as technology would allow.

The belated realization and discovery of the earthquake damage provided motivation for adaptability; keeping ones "cool" in the face of adversity and expecting the unexpected. Academic health centers are as complicated as small cities; issues arise on a daily basis although fortunately most of these are not transformative events.

In the end, the Northridge Earthquake presented an opportunity and need to construct three of the five new laboratory research buildings that would provide new seismically secure laboratory research space. Notably, all five were completed by 2008.

Another example of unwelcomed surprises occurred my very first weekend on the job. I was asked to meet with two county officials on a Saturday morning. They began the meeting by telling me that because of the heavy financial losses sustained by the county health-care system, the two UCLA affiliated county hospitals, Harbor UCLA Medical Center and Olive View UCLA Medical Center, may have to be closed. It was unlikely the county would electively close Los Angeles County USC Medical Center because of its pivotal positioning in the heart of a major underserved area of Los Angeles, as it was the largest facility of its kind in Los Angeles County. The Martin Luther King Medical Center was deemed untouchable since this facility was constructed as a result of promises made by the county and federal government to the residents of south Los Angeles following the Watts riots to ensure they would have a first-rate healthcare facility; an important necessity to provide proper healthcare for the underserved in the south Los Angeles area.

This was not one of those issues that required an immediate decision, but it mandated further adaptability because we had many faculty located at the Harbor and Olive View facilities; faculty who played a key role in teaching the medical students, in our post-graduate training programs teaching interns and residents, and in research. The UCLA faculty and the facilities were not only of fundamental importance to UCLA in their role in education and training, but the extent of the patient care mission was underappreciated by some county officials as these county facilities were needed in their own areas of South Bay and the San Fernando Valley because they provided critical services to the underserved. This problem directed me to understand the challenges of the Los Angeles County health system and who among the county officials I had to work closely with to achieve further understanding about the importance of the faculty and the facilities. The closures were averted when the Federal government and county worked through a financial plan that saved the facilities; another day, another crisis solved. Whatever I was doing (hopefully correctly) was a part of my subconscious and the instincts I had honed over a career in academic medicine.

As I reflect back on it now, these events helped steel me to participate in an extraordinary makeover of our entire academic health center that would catapult UCLA to a leadership position in the 21st century. My earlier experiences led to my ultimate reflections regarding the principles of leadership and the personal value system that every leader must possess. After all these years and reflecting on all that was accomplished no matter how difficult the task, it reaffirms that all things are indeed possible. Institutional leaders working with a great team and outstanding faculty can make a difference and trans-form an institution for the better. Even unfortunate, unpredictable and unwanted precipitating events have the potential to lead to won-derful outcomes.

I would now like to focus on the specifics of the two tables. Table One, *Personal Qualities for Successful Leadership: Personal Value System*, and Table Two, *Principles for Effective Leadership*. A *Personal Value System* has been defined as a set of principles or ideals that drive behavior. Your personal value system gives your life structure and purpose by helping to determine what is meaningful and important to you. It helps you express who you are and what you stand for, and it defines your character perhaps better than any other constellation of traits and principles. If you become disconnected from your values, it does not bode well for your perception as a leader in either an AHC or whatever organization you happen to be leading. The Personal Value System defines your very essence.

TABLE ONE

Personal Qualities for Successful Leadership: Personal Value System

- Honesty
- Having the highest integrity
- Having the highest ethical standards
- Keeping your promises
- Truthfulness
- Working hard and setting the standard
- Gravitas
- Treating everyone with respect
- Relating to people at all levels of the organization you lead
- Loyalty to the institution and its mission
- Having a sense of humor

On the website, www.essentiallifeskills.net/personalvaluesystem.html, there is an excellent discussion of the four categories of a *Personal Value System*. They are defined below:

Personal Values — Personal values are those traits that we see as worth aspiring to and that define our character.

Spiritual Values — The values that connect us to a higher power and give us a sense of purpose beyond our material existence.

Family Values — To love and care for those we are close to; our children, our parents, other family members, and our friends.

Career Values — The best use and expression of our talents and skills for the purposes of contributing to society and for monetary compensation.

The website also lists the values we as social beings find desirable. They include:

Integrity — Integrity is trustworthiness, honesty and uprightness of character. We value people of integrity because we know what to expect from them. We know they will act honorably and that they will do what they think is right. We want people with integrity as our friends, on our teams and in our organizations.

Respect — Respect is honoring the worth and dignity of all people. Those who respect others treat people with fairness and courtesy. They treat others the way they wish to be treated.

Loyalty — Loyalty is a commitment and faithfulness to a person or a cause. Those who are loyal to their family, friends, organizations and country and stand behind and support them during good times and bad times. They can be counted on to be there when the going gets difficult and to help out when the chips are down.

Responsibility — Those who accept responsibility are reliable, dependable and willing to take accountability for who they are and what they do. They believe it is their obligation to help others and to make a contribution to the society they live in.

It bears repeating that each of our own personal value systems is the essence of who you are and it will largely define your AHC or company or organization internally, the faculty and staff, and to the external world, i.e., patients, families, media, public officials and colleagues at other AHCs and their employees.

A few more comments regarding my personal value system seem worthwhile. I listed honesty, having the highest integrity, having the highest ethical standards, truthfulness and keeping your promises, working hard and setting the standard for work ethic, gravitas and having a sense of humor as being important as to how I lead my personal life and led my life as a leader at UCLA's Academic Health Center. If one contemplates this list or most any list of personal qualities contained in a personal value system, it becomes evident that the people who work within an AHC perceive that the leadership have strong personal value systems, whether they recognize it by that name or not. The personal value systems are the bedrock for faith and trust in the leader(s).

Honesty, integrity, truthfulness, keeping your promises, and the highest ethical standards should be everyone's goal no matter what organization you lead and no matter what other personal qualities are in your personal value system. Not only must the leader show these personal qualities but so must those leaders who report to the overall leader. It is important that the organization be positioned clearly on the side of zero tolerance when institutional honesty and integrity are violated by the leaders or by others. AHCs themselves are the size of small cities and towns; for example, UCLA's AHC consists of approximately 12,000 employees and it is expected that occasionally some behavior does not reflect the image of integrity that we represent and violates our personal value system. How you manage episodes that threaten the image of an AHC in the community and beyond can easily define and/or destroy your leadership. Again zero tolerance and an open, truthful, responsive and responsible corrective plan must be disclosed and implemented. Once trust in you is broken, it is almost impossible for you to recapture the trust, faith and respect of the faculty, students and staff. The old axioms "honesty is the best policy," "keep your word" and "don't make promises you can't keep" are as true today as ever before.

I initially began to recognize that others focused on my personal value system during several events where I was being honored prior to my stepping down from my position as vice chancellor and dean. Two of my direct reports, who spoke about me and several others who were interviewed on the video played at my retirement dinner, mentioned my integrity and honesty. The speakers, Dr. David Feinberg, CEO of the hospital system and Dr. Alan Robinson, associate vice chancellor for Medical Sciences and executive associate dean of the David Geffen School of Medicine, recalled that on several occasions over the years when they sought my advice prior to making a difficult decision they were required to make, I responded "never be afraid to do the right thing." That, apparently, was very important advice to them in analyzing these decisions. I was very grateful that they had pointed this out to the audience and the emphasis on integrity and honesty; it was very special to me, my wife and family. As I mentioned earlier, your honesty, ethical values and integrity are the essence of who you are. In a later discussion about this book, Dr. Feinberg suggested that "never be afraid to do the right thing" would be a great title and I am grateful to him for that suggestion since it is hard enough to write a book, let alone come up with a good title.

Table Two lists the *Principles for Effective Leadership* that are no less important, although different from the qualities listed in the *Personal Value System*.

Principles for Effective Leadership

- Surround yourself with high quality achievers and acknowledge their successes
- Cornerstones of an effective leadership team include a first-rate hospital CEO, a chief operating officer for academic programs and chief financial officer
- Work ethic and passion
- Check your ego at the door
- Vision: Set the bar high
- Responsibility: "The buck stops here"
- Don't rush judgments or decisions
- Admit when you are wrong and change direction
- Adaptability to meet unexpected changes and events
- Keep your composure
- Never forget the underlying academic mission
- If, after you analyze an issue and remain undecided, go with your instincts honed by a career in academia
- Be aware of your place in the history of the institution
- Be available for students, residents and junior faculty
- Communicate and personalize yourself
- Recognize that the role of the dean is to fulfill the dreams of the faculty, staff and students

Each principle is important, but I would like to highlight a few.

Recruit the highest quality individuals for the leadership team

It is worth repeating what I stated in the preface that the leader's success or failure is heavily dependent on the success or failure of his/her team. I have no doubt that the success I had at UCLA was directly related to the quality of individuals recruited for the team. Therefore, it is imperative that the leader recruit and retain the best people. They should be a blend of youth, experience and high energy, and dedicated to fulfilling the vision and achieving organizational success. They must share your personal value system. Do not micromanage your team. The team members are of high quality and they also have personal dreams and aspirations. They want to accomplish good things and it is necessary and appropriate for you to publicly acknowledge their successes on behalf of the organization. As leader you must provide the atmosphere and environment for them to thrive and they need you to provide them necessary mentorship.

When surveying the complex organizational structure of the leader's team, including the various deans and chairpersons, there emerges a clear need for the following special cornerstone appointments on the leadership team: an especially talented CEO of the hospital or hospital system; a first-rate academician/administrator to serve as chief operating officer for the School of Medicine, who is very close to the leader and looked upon as speaking for the leader in meetings, and a strong chief financial officer. All must have a passion for the academic mission. Another necessity is a strong chairperson(s) who can develop a cohesive chair group, shares the leader's broad vision for the institution and works well with the leader.

Work Ethic and Passion

The leader of an AHC should be someone who is passionate about carrying out the multitude of duties required to do leadership in the AHC and who is willing to give the time and effort required to achieve the goals set in the vision statement. The leader should have a sense of excitement in coming to work and being filled with pleasure and purpose for the job, i.e., a positive and personal adventure. Dr. Steven B. Sample, the former president of the University of Southern California, in his book *The Contrarians Guide to Leadership* would suggest this to mean that you are not "being" the leader you are "doing" the leader.

Ego

When you are the leader of an AHC, an axiom to remember is you should "check your ego at the door." You must learn that in many ways being a leader is a thankless job because most faculty and staff don't realize how difficult and complicated the day-to-day tasks associated with being a leader of a large organization are.

Vision

Keep your focus on a well-thought-out vision for the AHC and the goals you have set for the institution. With the passage of time, you will achieve milestones of accomplishments; gratification and satisfaction will follow. Set the bar high for your vision; you want to be the very best you can be in what you do. Although all AHCs are not equal in what they can do, in general, you should demand excellence in patient care, education, training and research. Also, be aware there is an abundance of "background noise" in any complicated leadership position that can be very distracting. You must learn to stay focused, ignore the noise and remember the main points of your vision.

Operating Style

You as a leader are dependent on the success of your direct reports to complete the goals you have set. You must provide the atmosphere and conditions as well as mentorship for them to succeed.

Composure

Always keep your composure. Be mindful of your place as the inspirational leader of the organization. When the going gets tough, the faculty and staff will look to you.

Responsibility

Responsibility for events, good and bad, falls on your shoulders. Remember another axiom "the buck stops here."

Finances

Manage the finances in a prudent manner and ensure you have adequate reserves to invest in new programs and to recruit and retain the best physicians and staff. Dean Sherman Mellinkoff, who served twenty-four years as dean of the UCLA School of Medicine (1962-1986), gave me my best advice when I was new to my duties, he said, "Jerry, your main job as dean is to fulfill the dreams of the faculty." In an AHC I would expand that to include students and staff. Everyone has a stake in the AHC and they deserve a chance to develop their talents in a well-managed financial institution.

In financial management, you have to spend to succeed. Just ensure you can afford it and make certain it is the right amount to spend for the right person or program. New programs should be accompanied by a business plan overseen by your chief financial officer.

Adaptability

You must be adaptable to change. Most every year there is something to be categorized as a major change in the environment; it is unusual for an AHC to operate continually under stable conditions.

Admit when you are wrong and change decisions and directions when necessary.

Communication

As the leader of a large organization, you must have a communication strategy. Everyone has an interest and share in the success of the AHC. There are many ways to communicate and different ones work for different people. There are online communications, general faculty meetings, bulletins, face-to-face meetings with small groups and attending department meetings once a year. At Merck I learned the power of face-to-face meetings; periodically, we were instructed to meet with our divisions and present ourselves for open questioning by the group, which included both scientists, physicians and staff. These meetings were well attended, unlike most general faculty meetings in academia. Being visible to the faculty and staff is one of the most important things you can do. Everyone in a large organization needs to be informed in order to understand our challenges and problems, as well as our successes.

Judgments and Decisions

Don't rush judgments or decisions; always remember there is time to think. There are very few problems that require such a rapid solution that you're prevented from thoroughly discussing the issue. Most issues are neither black nor white, a lesson you learn very quickly; there are least two sides to every story. Dr. Sample would recommend that you "think gray."

Finally, if you study an issue for a long period of time and cannot reach a comfortable decision, go with your instincts, those that were honed in your many years in academia. AHCs are a combination of academics and business and sometimes they are at variance. One of the major benefits for having AHCs is to broaden and strengthen the academic mission and to provide an environment that is favorable for translational research.

As you consider these principles, you will find most are also adaptable to a company or any type of organization or institution. The *Personal Value System* and the *Principles for Effective Management* hold true for a university, a corporation or a small business.

CHAPTER FOUR

THE FIRST FACULTY MEETING AND THE FIRST YEAR

In early 1979 when I was a faculty member at the University of Miami School of Medicine and would shortly be leaving to become chairman of medicine at the University of Pittsburgh School of Medicine, I had a meeting with the late Dr. William Harrington, who at that time was chairman of medicine at the University of Miami. During the conversation about the task facing me at the University of Pittsburgh and knowing that Pittsburgh's Department of Medicine had fallen on hard times, Dr. Harrington told me that he would like to offer one piece of advice that had served him well in his life as an academic administrator. He said, "Prepare for the job thoroughly before arriving on the scene full-time and lay out your plans for moving Pittsburgh's Department of Medicine ahead as rapidly as possible." He also said, "What you achieve in the first year of your tenure is often the legacy by which people will assess you and your leadership in the years ahead." I took his advice because of my respect for him and for his accomplishments at the University of Miami. As I quickly discovered at the University of Pittsburgh, it was the best advice anyone could have given me. The leadership at the University of Pittsburgh was business-oriented, wanted results and as quick a turnaround of the department as possible. They were appreciative of my approach to rebuilding the Department of Medicine and what I accomplished in the first year. The accomplishments included creating the first practice plan for the Department of Medicine; eliminating the financial deficit that had dire negative effects on the Department's growth and development; completing a number of key recruitments, including several excellent division chiefs; restoring morale of the faculty and house staff; initiating plans to build relationships throughout the campus and helping to strengthen the clinical services of the hospital.

When musing about the past, I recognize that I implemented the same strategy when I was recruited to UCLA to head UCLA's Medical Sciences. When I completed three months of concentrated study and analysis of the strengths and weaknesses at UCLA, I felt I had a grasp of the issues facing UCLA's Academic Health Center and how I could redirect and reenergize the major components of the Academic Health Center, i.e., the School of Medicine, the UCLA Medical Center and UCLA's Neuropsychiatric Hospital and the Faculty Practice Group.

The same strategy was even more effective than at Pittsburgh because the Medical Sciences at UCLA were a much bigger stage and much more was at stake.

By the end of the first year at UCLA, I succeeded in implementing a number of changes including numerous personnel changes; recruited several new department chairs; initiated the administrative process to create several new departments including Urology, Neurobiology, Family Medicine and Human Genetics; appointed a new chief of the Jonsson Comprehensive Cancer Center; completed the recruitment of a distinguished chief of pediatrics and began to demonstrate the fund-raising ability no one, including myself, knew I had. I asked Leslie and Susan Gonda, two wonderful individuals and philanthropists who were great supporters of UCLA, for $45 million to fund the construction of a research building which would be named the Gonda (Goldschmied) Neuroscience and Genetics Research Center. That research building would be the home of the new Department of Human Genetics and the site for the Brain Research Institute, the central organization that served as the coordinating body for Neuroscience on the entire UCLA campus. I also worked with the Department of Neurology to complete the funding for construction of the Ahmanson Lovelace Brain Imaging Building.

Years later one of our distinguished department chairs said to me, when we were reminiscing about my tenure at UCLA, that everyone knew "I meant business" when I started at full speed to make positive changes. In that vein while rummaging through the files a few months before starting to write this book, I unexpectedly found a copy of my talk at the first faculty meeting I held one month after I started full-time at UCLA. The presentation initiated and demarcated the steps we would be taking to enable UCLA's medical sciences to move forward again and take its rightful place as one of the great academic health centers in the United States. When you read the presentation you will notice little attention in my remarks discussing the Northridge Earthquake and its damaging effects on the medical sciences; the reports surfaced months later and the severity of the effects of the quake had not yet been established at UCLA. Nevertheless, despite the previously cited impact on the job description and my life at UCLA as vice chancellor and dean, everything mentioned in the presentation was completed; some sooner, some later. (See Appendix One)

The success I had implementing Dr. Harrington's advice is worthy of note in the context of leadership in large organizations like AHCs. The strategy worked well for me but it is clearly not for everyone nor is it appropriate for every situation a leader inherits when one assumes the leadership of a large organization. However, in this specific instance, I sensed a malaise within the medical sciences that was impairing our mission and keeping the organization from fully developing relationships with other schools on the UCLA campus especially the College of Letters and Sciences. My full team was not in place and I believe the decision to move forward decisively was the correct one.

In thinking back to the beginning of my tenure at UCLA, I am reminded of the classic book by Stephen R. Covey, *The 7 Habits of Highly Effective People*, a perennial best seller that has become one of the leadership bibles. The strategy espoused by Harrington was in reality an early version of Covey's analysis a decade later. In particular it is a model for Covey's first three habits, "Be Proactive," "Begin with the End in Mind," and "Put First Things First." Below, I have extracted the essence of these habits in order to better understand the concept of leadership.

Habit 1 Proactive people focus their efforts in the Circle of Influence. They work on the things they can do something about. The nature of their energy is positive, enlarging and magnifying, causing their Circle of Influence to increase.

Habit 2 To begin with the end in mind means to start with a clear understanding of your destination. It means to know where you're going so that you better understand where you are now and so that the steps you take are always in the right direction. Covey makes a clear distinction that "leadership is not management; that management has a bottom line focus." Habit 2 is also "the ability to envision, to see the potential, to create with our minds what we cannot at present see with our eyes."

Habit 3 Is effective self management characterized by "the ability to make decisions and choices and to act in accordance with them. It is the ability to act rather than to be acted upon." Covey believes that "effective management is putting first things first and that leadership decides what 'first things' are, while management is the discipline to carrying it out."

Clearly all three habits are interrelated and important qualities for all leaders. In the next chapter, I devote considerable time to another of Covey's concepts, the Emotional Bank Account, because I consider it a fundamental building block of leadership.

Before we move to Chapter Five, I will briefly summarize the substance of my remarks made to the UCLA faculty when I took the position as vice chancellor for Medical Sciences and dean of the David Geffen School of Medicine; Appendix One contains the complete unedited text of the presentation.

HIGHLIGHTS OF PRESENTATION TO THE FACULTY

- The first part of the faculty meeting was devoted to a presentation of the new governance structure, the reporting lines and my broad responsibilities. I also made a pledge to streamline the organization, make it more efficient and not create a bureaucracy, and reviewed the initiatives undertaken in the first month to implement the new organizational structure.

- The relationship between the hospital system and the medical school, and the hospital system and the Faculty Practice Group, and my plans and philosophy for implementing the changes needed to restore harmony and unity to Medical Sciences in a very difficult environment in California.

- The current state of the budget and my philosophy regarding the utilization of resources was addressed; I outlined the need for a major effort directed at fund-raising in order to develop new programs, new laboratory facilities, renovations of all the laboratories, endowed chairs, and other new buildings.

- I reviewed the status of recruiting for new chairpersons of the departments for Pediatrics, Pathology, Anatomy and Neurobiology, Surgery, the director of the Jonsson Comprehensive Cancer Center and development of a new Department of Human Genetics.

- The techniques I would employ to foster communications in this time of great change for UCLA's medical sciences.

- I provided my preliminary plans to providing much needed resources for the basic sciences.

- In the area of medical student education, I outlined my concerns about rising student fees, the need to enhance the numbers of our students entering careers in academic medicine, the need for enhancing the diversity of our faculty to provide appropriate mentors for our very diverse student body and the imperative for curriculum change.

The hour long presentation ended with a discussion of the relationships with our affiliates and their importance to our overall mission.

At the conclusion of this first faculty presentation, I thought I had made the desired impact; I had communicated a compelling rationale required for initiating change and I had shown that I possessed the energy, work ethic, determination and vision to successfully achieve our goals.

CHAPTER FIVE

"GOOD MORNING, HOW ARE YOU TODAY?"

In Steven Covey's *The 7 Habits of Highly Effective People*, he proposed the concept of an Emotional Bank Account which he likened to a financial bank account because we make deposits into it, build up reserves and make withdrawals when we need to. It's a fascinating concept. He uses the term "Emotional Bank Account" as a metaphor that describes the amount of trust that's been built up in a relationship. It is the feeling of safeness you have with another human being. If the leader makes deposits into an Emotional Bank Account through courtesy, kindness, honesty, and keeping his/her commitments to you, the leader builds up a reserve. Your trust toward the leader becomes higher, and the leader can call upon that trust many times if he or she needs to. The leader can even make mistakes and that trust level, that emotional reserve, will compensate for it. When the balance in the Emotional Bank Account is high, communication is easy, instant and effective. But if the leader has a habit of showing discourtesy, disrespect, cutting you off, overreacting, ignoring you, becoming arbitrary, betraying your trust, threatening you or playing little tin god in your life, eventually the Emotional Bank Account becomes overdrawn. The trust level gets very low and the leader loses support of the person or persons working in the organization.

Covey suggests there are six major deposits that build the Emotional Bank Account.

1. **Understanding the Individual**

   "Really seeking to understand another person is probably one of the most important deposits you can make, and it is the key to every other deposit." He then says, "To make a deposit, what is important to another person must be as important to you as the other person is to you. ... By accepting the value he places on what he has to say, you show an understanding of him that makes a great deposit."

2. **Attending to the Little Things**

   "The little kindnesses and courtesies are so important. Small discourtesies, little unkindnesses, little forms of disrespect make large withdrawals. In relationships, the little things are the big things."

3. Keeping Commitments

"Keeping a commitment or a promise is a major deposit; breaking one is a major withdrawal. In fact, there's probably not a more massive withdrawal than to make a promise that's important to someone and then not come through. The next time a promise is made, they won't believe it. People tend to build their hopes around promises, particularly promises about their basic livelihood."

4. Clarifying Expectations

"The cause of almost all relationship difficulties is rooted in conflicting or ambiguous expectations around roles and goals. We can be certain that unclear expectations will lead to misunderstanding, disappointment and withdrawals of trust. The deposit is to make the expectations clear and explicit in the beginning. This takes a real investment of time and effort upfront, but it saves great amounts of time and effort down the road."

5. Showing Personal Integrity

"Personal integrity generates trust and is the basis of many different kinds of deposits. Lack of integrity can undermine almost any other effort to create high trust accounts." Covey further states "integrity includes but goes beyond honesty. Honesty is telling the truth — in other words, *confirming our words to reality*. Integrity is *confirming reality to our words* — in other words, keeping promises and fulfilling expectations."

6. Apologizing Sincerely When You Make a Withdrawal

"When we make withdrawals from the Emotional Bank Account we need to apologize and we need to do it sincerely. Great deposits come in the sincere words: 'I was wrong.' 'That was unkind of me.' 'I showed you no respect.' 'I gave you no dignity, and I'm deeply sorry.' 'I embarrassed you in front of your friends and I had no call to do that.'"

With that introduction to Covey's concept of an Emotional Bank Account, I would like to provide some context to a real life situation at UCLA that is an excellent example of the concept of an Emotional Bank Account.

By nature I'm a gregarious person. Wherever I've been in my career, I have always made it a point to say good morning to the office staff and to inquire about their health, their family or some event that is special to them. I did the same for the various direct reports located in the vice chancellor/dean suite and faculty and staff I encountered in the hallways, cafeteria, etc. At the end of the day, for those who remained in the dean's office, my salutation was usually "good night" or "have a good evening." To be quite frank, I never really thought of what I was accomplishing by saying good morning or good night on a regular basis as being anything special on my part, it just seemed the natural thing to do. When the time came to step down after fifteen years from my position of vice chancellor for Medical Sciences and dean of the David Geffen School of Medicine at UCLA, Dr. Fawzy, one of the senior associate deans, said to me one morning the week before I stepped down, how much it meant to him to hear my good mornings in the suite including those directed at him. He had only been a senior associate dean for a year or so and previously thought from a distance that the atmosphere in the dean's office was probably cold and impersonal. He said his perception was incorrect. He also told me others in the office felt the same way about these little courtesies, acts of respect and friendship, which were much appreciated.

I can now recall from a different perspective the impact I had on their day to day working lives in the context of a metaphorical individual Emotional Bank Account; all this time I was, in actuality, making deposits into our respective Emotional Bank Accounts. Finally the day came when I had to make a "withdrawal" — although at that time I was still unaware of such a concept because it had been 20 years since I had read *The 7 Habits of Highly Effective People* and whatever retention of its concepts I had was lost long ago. In the summer of 2009, the president of the University of California and regents were forced to implement drastic cuts to the budget of the University of California system because the state of California was running a severe deficit. Salaries were cut for all employees, including the staff and vice chancellor/dean's office. I, and others, tried to have this decision rescinded for the affected staff, to no avail. I felt that the cut should not take place at the lower end of the salary scale only on those of us at high levels, since the impact on the state budget would be relatively minor but the impact on staff would be profound. I talked to each of the employees and said I was sorry; it wasn't fair to them because they really couldn't afford it, especially in this economy. All, however, were determined to get through this and one (Ms. Mia McGill) said to me, "We all have a job to do here, Dr. Levey, and we are all in this situation together." Despite the pain, they understood what was at stake; they persevered and made it through the year. I was very proud of her and the entire dean's office team.

After rereading Covey's book, I realized I had made numerous deposits into their individual Emotional Bank Accounts and they had enough trust in me to accept their cut in pay and yet my reserves of trust remained intact. Unknowingly I had fulfilled the second rule for a major deposit in the Emotional Bank Account by simply saying "good morning," smiling, being respectful and caring; I was attending to the little things and "in a relationship the little things are the big things."

I also fulfilled the sixth rule of deposits in the Emotional Bank Account "when making a withdrawal, apologize sincerely." This is an important message for leadership and therefore this seems a necessary chapter in the book about leadership. Every leader in an Academic Medical Center whether it is the dean, hospital CEO, department chair, etc., has to pay attention to the little things because they are in actuality the big things in life.

Certain principles of leadership or management relate to people at all levels in the organization, an important one being, treating everyone with respect. All faculty and staff want to believe they have a leader who can relate to them, who cares about them, who will give a nod or a smile in the morning, who might even get to know them and their family. This personalization of a relationship with your team and the faculty and staff is the kind of action that makes the organization special and that creates the environment that leads to a sense of togetherness, teamwork and focus on the organizational goals and a spirit of camaraderie. It bears repeating, the "little things are the big things" in life.

CHAPTER SIX

DECISIONS, DECISIONS, DECISIONS

Decision making is one of the most important functions for the leader of an organization whether it is an AHC or another type of institution or business. The first decision any leader has to make is what I call a decision about the decisions. That is, how to balance what are the most important decisions that directly affect the greater organization with other less important decisions which are, nevertheless, operationally important on a daily basis. Specifically, the leader has to resolve the question of how much decision making to relegate to him- or herself and how much to the direct reports? How does the leader stay informed when he or she is not the primary decision maker for an issue? It was my practice to relegate to my direct reports wide ranging latitude for decision making because they knew their specific areas, in many instances, better than I. However, I expected to be briefed on decisions they considered to be important *before* the decision was finalized, in case it was an issue that would affect the overall organization. They needed to recognize that I might request additional study and consideration.

The bottom line, however, is that the leader cannot be involved with most of the decisions because there are too many that have to be made on a daily or weekly basis. The key for success is having all of the leader's direct reports be totally aware of the vision and goals for the organization; to agree and espouse the same vision and goals; and be perfectly attuned to the leader's personal value system and management goals. Before we discuss the areas for which the leader must make the final decisions, I would like to quote a passage from the "Old Testament" describing an interaction between Moses and Moses' father-in-law, Jethro, the priest of Midian, found in Exodus 18:14 -27.

> *When Moses' father-in-law saw all that he did to the people, he said: "What is this thing that thou doest to the people? Why sittest thou thyself alone, and all the people stand about thee from morning unto even?" And Moses said unto his father-in-law: "Because the people come unto me to inquire of God; when they have a matter, it cometh unto me; and I judge between a man and his neighbor, and I make them know the statutes of God, and His laws." And Moses' father-in-law said unto him "The thing that thou doest is not good. Thou will surely wear away, both thou and this people that is with thee; for the thing is too heavy for thee; thou are not able to per-*

formeth thyself alone. Hearken now unto my voice, I will give thee counsel, and God be with thee: be thou for the people before God, and bring thou the causes unto God. And thou shalt teach them the statutes and the laws and shalt show them the way wherein they must walk, and the work they must do. Moreover thou shalt provide out of all the people able men, such as fear God, men of truth, hating unjust gain; and place such over them to be rulers of thousands, rulers of hundreds, rulers of fifties and rulers of ten. And let them judge the people at all seasons; and it shall be, that every great matter they shall bring unto thee, but every small matter they shall judge themselves; so shall they make it easier for thee and bear the burden with thee. If thou shalt do this thing, and God command thee so, then thou shalt be able to endure, and all this people also shall go to their place in peace." So Moses hearkened to the voice of his father-in-law, and did all that he had said. And Moses chose able men out of all Israel, and made them heads over the people, rulers of thousands, rulers of hundreds, rulers of fifties, and rulers of tens. And they judged the people at all seasons: the hard causes they brought unto Moses, but every small matter they judged themselves. And Moses let his father-in-law depart and he went his way into his own land.

This was probably the first recorded discussion of decision making and the governance structure of a large organization of approximately 600,000 Hebrews, navigating their way across the Sinai Desert to the Promised Land to be known as Israel. The wisdom in this discussion some 3,000 years ago and its applicability and similarity to modern organizations is amazing.

Since I read scripture on a nightly basis, I recognized the importance of this the first time I read the passage after assuming the leadership post at UCLA. The message gets to the heart and soul of a fundamental principle of management. Jethro's recommendation was that Moses depend more on his "team" so he could function more effectively as the leader of the Israelites.

My Jethro, a man named Willie, cleaned the dean's suite each night. During my first year, before I had my management team in place, I would see him from 7:30 to 8:00 p.m. after my typical 12 to 14 hour day and he said to me one night in his soft southern drawl, "Dr. Levey, time to go home; you're going to burn out." When I had completed my team recruitment, I took his sage advice; he was a wise person and I am grateful that he cared about my health and well-being.

Here are specific areas I consider important enough to fall within the leader's purview; items the leader should have the final say in the decision.

BUDGET:
In an AHC the core issue is the responsible management and provision of financial support using the resources available to maintain the

excellence of the academic mission. Funds from all corners of the enterprise must flow to the School of Medicine for the academic mission because ultimately all units of the enterprise, including the hospital(s) and practice plans, are the beneficiaries of high quality physicians and scientists that result in the highest quality patient care, the best teaching of medical students, residents, interns, staff, the highest patient satisfaction, and a positive impact on the community in which the AHC is located.

RECRUITMENT AND RETENTION:

The responsible and prudent flow of funds also requires the availability of financial support to recruit clinical and basic science chairs, sometimes in partnership with the hospital and the relevant department, and to recruit and retain key clinicians and scientists.

Each member of the team of direct reports must carry out the key functions of the broader organization especially those that pertain to administrative functions that sub-serve the faculty, departments, hospital(s), students and staff. The act of recruiting direct reports (depending on the governance structure of the AHC) should include the hospital CEO. Recruitment is a function of great importance to the entire organization because of the role one is recruited for. The hospital must be kept financially strong and vibrant; the leader and the hospital CEO must be partners who work well together; and the CEO must understand and be in accord with the academic mission and the leader's goals.

STRATEGIC ALLIANCES, ACQUISITIONS AND CONSTRUCTION OF NEW BUILDINGS:

This category includes hospitals and any school of medicine with which the AHC wishes to affiliate for academic or clinical reasons including educational and research affiliations and international alliances that subserve the broad mission of an AHC. For example, UCLA acquired the Santa Monica Medical Center in August 1995 and consummated a strategic alliance with Los Angeles based Orthopaedic Hospital in 1998. From 1994 to 2008, UCLA's AHC undertook a vast building program following the Northridge Earthquake including construction of the new Ronald Reagan UCLA Medical Center completed in 2008, the Santa Monica/UCLA and Orthopaedic Hospital to be completed in 2011 or 2012, and five research buildings all completed between 1997 and 2008.

FUND-RAISING AND DONOR SATISFACTION:

Fund-raising and donor satisfaction serves the broader institutional goals. For example, donors contribute to the new hospitals, research buildings, programs and endowed chairs, all of which benefit the broader organization. Donors are a critical source of both restricted and unrestricted funds and are a lifeline for the academic and clinical programs. The leader of the AHC must have the direct, hands-on leadership role of this area. It is critical to the budget of any AHC.

Nevertheless, despite this impressive list of areas which the leader must have final decision, the leader must also recognize that any decision, large or small, or whether or not it was assigned to a direct report's area of responsibility will ultimately reflect on the leader, whether it be good or bad. As the old saying goes and it cannot be emphasized too much, "the buck stops here" and your desk is where the buck stops, therefore, be careful, listen to others' opinions, think the issues through but don't be timid, and be open to making bold decisions when consistent with your goals.

Another observation to be aware of is that the outcome of some decisions are immediate; but some are not seen for many years and you have to be patient. For example, when I arrived on the scene in Los Angeles, the UCLA Medical Center was in the midst of negotiations with UniHealth America to buy the Santa Monica Hospital, as UniHealth was in the process of selling the hospitals that it owned. These were difficult times for hospitals in California because of a severely recessed economy and a market place that was being seriously eroded by managed care, which resulted in decreased reimbursement rates. Regarding the sale of Santa Monica Hospital to UCLA in the late spring of 1995, the agreement on the purchase was approaching a conclusion. Two key figures at the UCLA Medical Center, who were most important to the negotiating process for the purchase, decided to leave UCLA. I was left to make the fateful decision in one week or the agreement to purchase would likely be terminated. After only nine months or so on the job, I experienced great apprehension and undertook a cram course to expand my knowledge base as soon as possible for this purchase. I decided to approve the purchase of the Santa Monica Hospital as it was in our best interest for several reasons, although not without risk. Expanding a program in woman's health was part of my vision for UCLA's greater academic and clinical mission, and Santa Monica Hospital had an exceptionally strong obstetrics and gynecologic presence in Santa Monica and the Westside of Los Angeles; Santa Monica Hospital also had one of our nation's extraordinary programs, The Rape Treatment Center. In addition, the department of medicine at UCLA was developing a large primary care network with the generous support of the CEO of the UCLA Medical Center and many of the physicians in the network were linked with the Santa Monica Hospital. A Santa Monica/UCLA Medical Center, in our estimation, would serve as part of this regional network since most of the patients presumably would be hospitalized in either Santa Monica/ UCLA or the tertiary care oriented UCLA Medical Center.

Even after the decision was made, it proved to be very difficult to develop the linkages between the community, UCLA, and the physicians; neither was UCLA's position enhanced in the market place. The hospital also continued to lose money. Over the years that followed, my positive feelings that all would be well and the hospital would be profitable alternated with grim foreboding for the financial health of the Santa Monica UCLA Medical Center. On many occasions, I felt I had made the wrong decision in approving the purchase of the hospital. However, the regrets I had, slowly but surely, lessened in recent years and since

2008, the hospital has been profitable, thanks to a number of initiatives, and is now playing a key role in our clinical presence in the community. These initiatives included an alliance with Orthopaedic Hospital of Los Angeles to form the Santa Monica UCLA Medical Center and Orthopaedic Hospital; the seismic renovation of the hospital to meet all earthquake standards and to have a new hospital rising from the old hospital that would position us better in the market place and be more attractive to patients; the primary care network was streamlined over the years and became more effective; most of the clinical departments led by the Department of Medicine's yeoman work were engaged in transferring clinical programs to the Santa Monica/UCLA Medical Center from the new Ronald Reagan UCLA Medical Center; and relations between UCLA and the community physicians improved. The consensus opinion regarding this hospital purchase if it had been measured over the short term would have been that it was an abject failure, however, patience and the most precious commodity, time, as well as the adaptation of the School of Medicine clinical departments to more fully and completely build services at Santa Monica/UCLA Medical Center and Orthopaedic Hospital, were decisive. Now, anyone who studied this purchase of the hospital and the key role it is now playing would conclude that our organization and its leader made the correct long-term decision. It was a special sense of satisfaction and joy to know that our entire organization pulled together and made our decision the *best* decision and helped establish UCLA's medical services more firmly in the Westside of Los Angeles.

Ten Principles for Effective Decision Making

As I have thought about what I have learned in the area of decision making, I put forth the following ten principles:

1. AHCs are complex organizations that have both a business and an academic mission. They are constantly in delicate balance and decision making must take both into account.

2. When in doubt about a decision, despite thorough review and analysis, go with your instincts honed in a career in academic medicine.

3. Making sound decisions requires the leader to be not only aware of the complex mission but what has made the AHC successful. The history and tradition of the institution means a great deal; academic excellence and the core missions of education, research and patient care, and the maintenance of the highest ethical standards are the infrastructure of good decision making.

4. Most decisions should be based on thorough analysis and not be done in haste. To prevent "deferred" decisions which could prove harmful to the organization, there should be time limits for a decision.

5. There is always time to think.

6. A willingness to change and adopt new ideas is a worthy undertaking but only if it is compatible with what the institution represents.

7. Decisions pertaining to overtly problematic issues, such as

personnel performance, inappropriate behavior, etc., need to be addressed. Although decisions may be difficult, the problem usually doesn't resolve itself with time and indecision. It is better to face the issue and reach a resolution. However, the leader must recognize that you can't rush to judgment. Personnel issues require special attention to due process and fairness.

8. In decisions regarding business opportunities, the need for up-to-date accurate data is paramount. This is easier said than done in a medical environment that is generally unstable and subject to economic and political pressures, and unknown effects of the continual changes in the healthcare system.

9. The direct reports of the leader need mentoring, responsibility and a quality learning experience to assist in their career development. Decision making skills are a necessity for growth in leadership skills.

10. "Never be afraid to do the right thing," was one of my responses to several of my direct reports when they asked for my opinion on decisions that were theirs to make and they were uncertain of the ultimate outcome of their decision. Even if that yardstick results in an unpopular decision, the decision must be put into the context of ethics and institutional and personal integrity. On that basis, it will always be the "right decision."

To conclude this chapter, there are many important decisions that have to be made by a leader during the course of any given year at any AHC or organization. I am certain that the number of significant decisions I had to make in my fifteen years as leader of UCLA's Medical Sciences numbered in the hundreds, if not thousands. I have thought long and hard about the single most important class of decisions I have had to make during that time, and I am convinced they were the decisions regarding personnel.

I had about forty direct reports, all of whom played key roles in establishing and maintaining the many strengths and successes of UCLA's medical enterprise. If you include faculty retentions and recruitments in which I became personally involved, the number reaches several hundred. The leader must excel in this function because team building and having an "A team" is fundamental to success; in fact, if you don't build an outstanding leadership team, chances for success will be limited. An "A team" requires an outstanding chief operating officer (executive associate dean), chief financial officer, chief executive officer of the hospital system, chief operating officer of the hospital system, associate and assistant deans, associate vice chancellors, department chairs, chiefs of major centers and programs — variations to this model will depend on the size and complexity of the AHC. Most of the personnel that I have had the pleasure to appoint at UCLA have been highly successful. When misjudgments occur, and I certainly made some, they need to be rectified either by education and counseling, or termination from the administrative responsibilities. The organization is only as strong as its weakest link. Mistakes in hiring need to be minimized because recruitments are time consuming, costly and the wrong person can disrupt the team's esprit and accomplishments. My advice would be to take the time to satisfy yourself that you have made the correct decision; vet candidates thoroughly and appoint the best search committees and or search firms; have your appropriate direct reports and outstanding, thoughtful faculty interview the candidates and provide the additional broadening of perspective; heed the interviewers' impressions. The end result is worth the effort.

CHAPTER SEVEN

FINANCIAL MANAGEMENT

Responsible and effective financial management of any organization is critical. This is the leader's responsibility and one must be constantly involved so as to understand the day-to-day financial issues that impact the organization. The question constantly arises: does the leader need to have a masters of business administration? The answer, in my estimation, is no. For instance, there has only been one US President, George W. Bush, who has had an MBA, and the President is in charge of the largest budget in the world. However, I want to state unequivocally at the outset that the key to first-rate financial management in any organization such as an AHC is to ensure that there are superior CFOs for both the medical school and the hospital. The CFOs must be able to meaningfully communicate between each other and with the respective leaders in the medical school and the hospital; they must share a concern for each unit of the AHC and commit to working together. I suppose I could end the chapter at this point, but I feel that defining a clear role for the leader is also necessary and important. Fulfillment of the mission and vision of the leader requires strong financial management as well as constant dialogue about that mission and goals, including new goals or missions that arise. This requires that the leader of an AHC must be involved with day-to-day financial issues. The academic mission is paramount; the leader must keep this essential thought at the forefront of everyone on the financial management team's mind. The leader must make it perfectly clear that the resources available are viewed as totally fungible and must be used to strengthen the education, training, research and clinical mission. It is the leader who will have to shoulder the blame if the school of medicine and hospitals are not properly nurtured. Keeping those options open maximizes the future ability for the hospital and medical school to be fiscally strong and for their success to be sustainable for the foreseeable future. Reserves need to be strengthened for the entire organization; unrestricted and restricted endowments need to be built and practices put in place to ensure their future growth. The leader, working in concert with the hospital CEO and/or the dean of the school of medicine (in the UCLA model, the leader is both dean and vice chancellor), needs to focus on building this platform of reserves and endowment to provide stability to the school and hospital, and particularly, to support the mission. As mentioned earlier, the leader has to ensure that the CFOs of the school of medicine and hospital work closely together and understand the goals regarding the academic mission and the need to direct resources where they are needed. In some AHCs, tension develops between the school and the hospital which is seriously counterproductive to the mission and, therefore, unacceptable; it is the leader who must ensure that any tension is quickly dissipated and problems corrected. Everyone also needs to understand the vulnerability and needs of the school of medicine and the vulnerability and needs of the hospital to further emphasize the requirement for a single mission, working in unison and having the same goals.

FINANCIAL RESOURCES AVAILABLE TO THE SCHOOL OF MEDICINE

(The percentages of items listed below vary depending upon each individual AHC and what specific parts of the mission they emphasize at a particular time.)

1. Direct and indirect costs from federal grants; especially the National Institutes of Health (NIH), the largest single provider of research support to schools of medicine and other federal agencies such as the National Science Foundation
2. Pharmaceutical industry support of clinical trials
3. Taxation of Practice Plan income
4. Tuition and fees
5. Federal, state and local contracts

6. Transfers from the hospitals to provide reimbursement to the medical school for clinical service chiefs who are generally school of medicine physicians; seed funds to start new clinical programs; recruitment and retention of key physicians and physician/scientists

7. Philanthropy

8. Interest from endowments and reserves

9. Scholarship funds

10. State support

SCHOOL OF MEDICINE VULNERABILITIES

1. Failure to build reserves and endowments over a broad range — from scholarship funds to operating resources for new programs, recruitments and retentions

2. Failure to provide proper support and oversight to ensure each of the medical school departments remain fiscally sound, totally functional and able to carry out the broader goals of the department

3. Failure to control expenses

4. Failure to provide modern teaching facilities and up-to-date research facilities

5. Failure to maximize cash intake — look for new sources of cash by increasing the flow of receivables; ensuring you are billing properly and not leaving money on the table

FINANCIAL RESOURCES AVAILABLE TO THE HOSPITAL

1. Patient reimbursement

2. Interest from reserves and endowment

3. Clinical trials

4. Direct costs from research grants (in most AHCs, grants are run through the school of medicine)

5. State and local contracts

6. Philanthropy

HOSPITAL VULNERABILITIES

1. Failure to develop and maintain secure cash reserves to protect the hospital during down periods in the marketplace; carries with it the threat of fiscal instability

2. Failure to maintain debt capacity to provide for facility upgrades, new construction and new equipment

3. Failure to continuously improve reimbursement for contracts

4. Failure to properly manage accounts receivables

5. Failure to develop endowments

6. Failure to be in a position to support new program development, recruitment and retention of key physicians

7. Failure of expense management

It is worth reiterating that the leader has the ultimate responsibility for securing the resources of the entire organization including the hospitals, school of medicine and practice plans despite some differences in needs; e.g., cash reserves (hospitals) and scholarship funding (school of medicine). It is the leader to whom the faculty will look to for appropriately running the economic "ship of state" and to provide the necessary funding to "fulfill their dreams." If you communicate in an honest way through the good times and bad, your Emotional Bank Account will sustain you. Hurricanes, earthquakes and major national recessions as causes of financial difficulty can be forgiven by faculty, students and staff and acknowledged with understanding and patience. Fiscal mismanagement will not be tolerated nor understood; and there will be appropriate demands for change from faculty, students and staff. The Emotional Bank Account will not save you. Fiscal mismanagement will be viewed as a failure of your *Personal Value System* and your stated Principles of Management (see Chapter Three). It cannot and should not occur. The leader must never forget that faculty, students and staff are very dependent on the leader for many reasons, but even more so when financial times are difficult.

The faculty, students and staff inherently want to be immune from the difficulties of financial management. Basically, they come to work and each day want to feel secure, that they have a special role and that their careers will be well-served by the institution. Faculty members want to be able to do their work, establish their roles within the university and nationally, to be rewarded with timely promotions and to be paid appropriately. The students want the best teaching and learning facilities; a topnotch hospital and faculty, who cares about them; and especially a devoted leader who cares about the quality of their experience and education. The staff who work at the medical school or hospital want jobs that are of interest and give them a sense of importance and fulfillment; the chance to "move up the ladder" to better positions; and to feel proud of the institution they work for. They also want to have the ease of mind that someone with integrity is in charge, that the various decisions made in the name of fiscal management will be for the benefit of the institution and will not, in any way, sully the reputation of the AHC.

Thus, the leader working with the chief financial officer(s) and other members of the team must do all that is humanly possible to avoid bad fiscal management; to ensure institutional economic health and the ability to plan and invest in research, education, new clinical programs; and to perform the necessary functions of recruitment and retention. Continuous financial planning to move the institution forward should be a goal of both the medical school and the hospital. The hospital and the school of medicine share the same mission. In fact, the hospital and school of medicine are interlocked; in general, the better the medical school does, the better the hospital does, and vice versa. Cooperation and cohesion of the two major subunits of the AHC manifest themselves by being better able to recruit the best physicians, scientists, nurses, staff and students. In addition, it also serves as an attractant to potential donors to financially strengthen the hospitals and the medical school. The better the fiscal management, the better the likelihood that the entire mission of the AHC will be able to be fulfilled. The leader should never permit the financial standing to slip; bad fiscal management leads to large deficits, paralysis in developing programs and fulfilling the mission of the institution. As a consequence, the leader is unintentionally not allowing the dreams of the faculty, students and staff to be fulfilled.

Long-term planning is a necessity, but difficult to do if the one, three and five year projections do not show appropriate sources of revenue for those long-term plans and instead new initiatives must be implemented to reverse the situation so long-term planning can take place. The main point is that the leader must recognize this early and receive the appropriate advice from the chief financial officer(s) to be able to reconcile this with his or her plans.

To simplify, in regards to the financial management arena, there is a very distinct role for the leader of an AHC to play; this is one of the most important areas for the leader to show interest, knowledge, enthusiasm, determination and good common sense. The leader is responsible for the entire family of faculty, students and staff, and it is a heavy responsibility to bear.

CHAPTER EIGHT

THE VISION, THE MISSION AND THE STRATEGIC PLAN

"If you don't know where you are going, chances are you'll end up somewhere else." – Yogi Berra

One of the most important things a leader must accomplish very early in his or her administration is the development of the vision statement. I felt it was necessary to incorporate and invigorate my philosophy about having an immediate impact on the organization which was described in Chapter Four. From my early meetings, I detected an urgency to deliver to faculty, staff and students a sense of the future challenges, goals and aspirations. Before I arrived full-time at UCLA, I considered it a priority to learn about the institution. I spent much of the summer and early fall talking with faculty, department chairs and other key individuals, becoming informed about the issues

that were foremost on their minds, including programmatic impera-
tives, strengths and weaknesses, and what would be fulfilling initiatives for the first five years of my tenure. At the end of this period, I
felt I was in synchrony with key faculty and was able to articulate a
vision statement. UCLA's medical sciences vision statement emphasized twelve areas to receive special attention in order to achieve first-
tier status as an AHC in the 21st century. The agenda would build on
the earlier successes of faculty and leadership since the inception of
the school in 1947. For example, cardiovascular disease and cancer
research as well as clinical care were thriving, well-respected locally
and nationally, and would continue to be emphasized. The following
areas needed attention (there were a mixture of administrative, clinical, research and development issues):

1. Implementation of a new governance structure

2. Neurosciences

3. Human Genetics

4. Geriatrics

5. Women's health

6. Men's health

7. Philanthropy

8. Community

9. Developing relationships with the Division of Life Sciences

10. Creation of new departments

11. New and innovative curriculum

12. Primary care network

This list became a mantra for speeches that I gave to multiple community organizations who invited me to speak about UCLA's medical sciences, at general faculty meetings and face-to-face meetings with every department in the school of medicine. I was deeply concerned with ensuring successful communication of the vision statement so that everyone was on the same page.

It became apparent that the vision statement was a "living" document subject to change, and with change usually comes delay, however, I was not expecting the accomplishments to come as quickly as they did producing much in the way of early success (see Chapter Four) and within the first five years, the following accomplishments occurred with regard to the specific initiatives delineated in the first vision statement:

1. The new governance structure for the medical sciences was successfully and fully implemented and the breech that occurred between the hospital and the medical school was rectified. It has been clearly delineated that the hospital system has an important role as a key partner of the school of medicine in nourishing the academic mission.

2. Neurosciences — Two new chairs were appointed; one for the Department of Psychiatry and Biobehavioral Sciences, and the other for the Department of Neurology. Construction was completed on the Ahmanson-Lovelace Brain Mapping Building. Plans were conceived and construction begun on a new neuroscience

research building. Funding for the new Gonda (Goldschmeid) Neuroscience and Genetics Research Building was made possible by a large gift from the donor; the building was completed in 1997 and serves as the home for the Brain Research Institute and the Department of Human Genetics.

3. The Department of Human Genetics was approved by the Faculty Senate; space was identified in the new building and an inaugural chair of the department recruited. Under the leadership of the late Leena Peltonen, a world figure in human genetics, the department enjoyed early success and continues today as a premier department.

4. Geriatrics — Geriatrics continued to thrive at a higher plane in terms of patient care and clinical research. Multiple departments are involved in the program. The Geriatric program has been consistently rated in top 5 in the United States; and in the *U.S. News and World Report* is frequently voted number one.

5. Woman's health programs were organized and were immeasurably helped by a large donation from Iris Cantor, a philanthropist interested in women's health. The clinic is now one of our busiest and is fully integrated with our Departments of Obstetrics and Gynecology and Internal Medicine. Several Center of Excellence grants were obtained through NIH.

6. Men's Health — the Division of Urology became the Department of Urology and has become a leading center for both cutting edge research and clinical care of prostate cancer, kidney cancer,

erectile dysfunction and disorders of the bladder.

7. Philanthropy more than quadrupled over a five year period.

8. Relationships were dramatically improved with the community and the School of Medicine was awarded the AAMC Community Service Award in 1998.

9. Developing close working relationships within the Division of Life Sciences in the College of Letters and Sciences was achieved within the first two years. Two departments of Microbiology and Immunology, one from the medical school and one from the college, were successfully merged. The dean of the Division of Life Sciences was appointed as an associate dean in the Medical School for joint programs between the Division and School of Medicine. Several new interdepartmental PhD programs were developed.

10. Starting in 1996, a complete makeover of the curriculum occurred that would better prepare our students for 21st century medicine.

11. The development of a primary care network by the Department of Medicine took about ten years to fully develop and refine, but within the first five years, it had already become a major clinical initiative for the department and for the UCLA Health System in its geographic market.

At the end of five years, it was already evident that the vision statement would need to be revisited. The updated vision statement most notably included plans for three new research buildings to provide seismically safe research space for scientists in the School of Medicine and construction of the new Ronald Reagan UCLA Medical Center. As you may remember, the old UCLA Medical Center had been irreparably damaged in the Northridge Earthquake in 1994. Also, the acquisition of the Santa Monica Hospital in 1995 enabled UCLA to develop the Santa Monica/UCLA Medical Center and Orthopaedic Hospital. That allowed UCLA to rebuild those hospitals so they are seismically safe; construction is due to be completed sometime in 2011–12. Other items that were added to the new vision statement included a concerted effort to have the UCLA School of Medicine endowed and named, a milestone achieved in 2002 following the extraordinary donation of $200,000,000 by David Geffen. Other philanthropy goals included securing at least one hundred new endowed chairs and markedly increased endowment for scholarships.

One further consideration when discussing vision statements is that many people are unsure of the precise difference between a vision statement, a mission statement and a strategic plan, especially the difference between the vision statement and the strategic plan. I will attempt to provide my view of what each is and hope to clarify any confusion.

Vision Statement

A good vision statement is more challenging than it seems at first blush since there are overlaps between the vision and mission statements, and a strategic plan. Nevertheless, to be direct and succinct, a vision statement must be all about the future direction(s) the leader wants to move the organization. A vision statement is probably the most important statement for the institution whether the organization is an AHC, a community hospital, multi-specialty clinic or a general healthcare business; and is one of the most important features of leadership because in it the leader clearly defines the direction for the future of the organization. In addition to establishing the goals and areas of interest, the vision statement ideally should provide inspiration and excitement; it must be doable, believable, and substantive to the audience you are trying to reach and demonstrate a concern for correcting specific weaknesses. The vision statement must be true to the Personal Value Scale of the individuals who make up the organization and be consistent with the institutional culture, values and traditions. If you don't have the appropriate goals and tone for the vision statement or can't communicate it clearly, I would remind you of the quote from Yogi Berra who said, *"If you don't know where you are going, chances are you'll end up somewhere else."* As with so many things on which Yogi opined, he was very wise.

To summarize, the vision statement is about the future, not about the present. The vision statement is a "living" statement that must be constantly amended with the changing needs of the organization.

Mission Statement

The mission statement is about the organization at the present time. The Mission Statement of the David Geffen School of Medicine is four fold: Research, Education, Patient Care and Public Service. These components are synergistic:

- Research creates knowledge about biologic science, human health and prevention, detection, and treatment of human disease
- Education disseminates that knowledge
- Patient care applies the knowledge
- Public service utilizes all three to benefit the community

The mission statement is, in effect, the purpose of the organization and the foundation of what the institution does.

Strategic Plan

The strategic plan is the implementation arm of the vision statement. The leader creates the vision of the organization; it is the management team that delineates the steps required to achieve the vision set out in the vision statement including resources needed and how to achieve the strategic aims. I want to emphasize that the strategic plan does not create the vision, the mission or the core values; it is focused on how to implement the plan delineated in the vision statement and, if possible, to provide needed reliable forecasting of the future.

The strategic plan is often difficult to implement. Strategic planning is expensive financially, especially if one relies heavily on consultants. The consultants can help with providing a structure for the strategic plan but basically the strategic plan will rise and fall with the commitment of leadership at all levels and the commitment of the faculty. The leader must clearly articulate the goals of the strategic plan and what you hope to achieve; therefore, the goals must be sharp, well defined and well thought out; the goals shouldn't be diffuse and overly broad. Remember the strategic plan is also costly in regard to faculty time, and if the constituents don't identify with and buy into the strategic plan, it will likely be relegated to the shelf and never be implemented.

This era of change characterized by healthcare reform and the financial environment of a stressed economy has served to make this a very challenging time for planning and the risk of erroneous forecasting higher than usual. Our turbulent and changeable economy makes it exceptionally difficult to do long-range planning for any organization, no less AHCs, even forecasting one to two years is a formidable challenge. Quoting another truism from Yogi Berra, *"It's tough to make predictions especially about the future."* At this time in history, he is right on target.

In summary, if the vision statement is worthwhile, it is worth the time and effort to implement the strategic plan well, by being aware of and avoiding the various obstacles inherent in the environment in which we are living.

CHAPTER NINE

RECRUITMENT AND RETENTION

The leader of an AHC or any major healthcare organization has a selective but important role in the area of recruitment and retention. For recruitment the leader needs to have the final say regarding any individual who will be on the organizational chart reporting to him or her. However, it is useful and desirable for the leader to have input from his or her other direct reports. In an AHC it is commonplace for the leader to be requested to interview a top candidate who some department or division of a department or program is anxious to recruit, someone with extraordinary potential to be a future leader or someone who has already reached the status of a leader in the field. Under the circumstances, your approval, your special insights and possible willingness to invest resources from the central administration can be decisive. An interview with the leader generally leaves an important positive impression upon the candidate who is being recruited.

In addition, successful and wise recruitment in all key areas is an important and worthwhile undertaking for the leader because it helps to maintain and/or enhance the traditions of excellence at the institution, and if the recruits do well, they will further enhance the reputation of the institution. Building excellence by wise recruiting also makes it easier to recruit other scientists and clinicians and helps to attract the finest medical, graduate and postdoctoral students. Furthermore, an enhanced reputation of the institution and having the finest clinicians is attractive to the public who will seek care at the hospital system and clinics, as these clinicians generally provide early access to the latest in medical advances. This in turn makes it easier to attract potential donors who provide important sources of income. Broad donor support starts a new source of revenue, which in turn enhances the reputation as well as the ability to recruit.

Similarly, a selective role can be played by the leader in retention issues which are commonplace in academic institutions. Reasons for retention usually focus on issues of salary; schooling for the candidates children; promotions or promotion acceleration; need for the faculty member to relocate to another area of the country to be closer to family and, of course, the opportunity of being offered an excellent position by a recruiting institution or organization who is competing with you for the candidate.

If the person you are trying to retain is a critical player in the research, education, or clinical arena for your AHC, the cost of trying to recruit a replacement will generally be more expensive than the retention package required to keep the faculty member from leaving. Given the economic turbulence characterized by the present environment, the cost could be prohibitive to replace the person who leaves. In the era in which we live, it is very expensive to train individuals and to nourish them during their early years as a faculty member or to recruit established scientists or clinicians. At UCLA we have made special efforts to retain our best and brightest at all faculty levels as well as to carefully select targeted recruitments.

For very special recruitments and retentions, it may be necessary to request that the chancellor or president of the University meet with them to try to have a positive effect on the person or persons being recruited or retained. Upon occasion, the chancellor or president may even provide some resources for someone who also impacts other departments on campus. It is also wise to involve the chairperson of the Governance Board of the institution, who may be effective in convincing the person being recruited or the retainee to accept our offer.

General Comments Regarding the Recruitment of Your Direct Reports

The recruitment of your direct reports is of critical importance to how you function. Basically, your success or failure as leader is dependent on their performance, since institutions like AHCs are very large and complex and you as leader cannot, by any stretch of the imagination, do it alone.

For everyone you appoint, you should aim high. You want people who are smart and talented. If you recruit highly intelligent individuals, they are usually fast learners and bring their own unique perspectives. It can be a source of great satisfaction to observe their development on the job. Other essential characteristics and qualities to look for during recruitment are youth, energy, vitality, hard workers and those who have excellent people skills. If your team has the above characteristics and the correct Personal Value Scale, the greater the chance that your vision will be carried out.

Responsibility to Your Reports

You have certain responsibilities you must fulfill as a leader to the people you recruit and report to you.

- The leader must ensure that the team grows and develops both individually and as a group. You should incorporate and utilize each person as a part of the team, someone who becomes familiar with all the issues and acquainted with the general goals, successes and problems of the organization.

- Prepare them for life in the organization after you. It is your responsibility to see that they develop independence and self-reliance.
- Any misadventures by your direct reports reflects badly on you and your team. It is your responsibility to know before they are appointed what their Personal Value Scale is and try to prevent problems before they start.
- In order to have an effective team, they cannot and should not be micromanaged. High quality, smart people generally do not function well when being micromanaged. The team leaders in the AHC must have the opportunity to show what they can do and be recognized for their skills and accomplishments. Like interns, residents and junior faculty, the team needs a learning experience.
- Criticism should be constructive and done in private; in contrast, the accomplishments of a direct report should be recognized publicly. Giving credit where credit is due is much appreciated.
- Career counseling is also a responsibility; you should be available to help with issues that involve career counseling.
- You have responsibility to guide them to promotions within the organization.
- Give them their environmental and intellectual space in which to work and function and you will be more than rewarded by

their performance.

- If warranted by a poor performance review, a direct report who does not function up to expectations at some point will require remediation, and if that fails, termination may be necessary. It is very hard to keep some team members from failing, but in a large, complex organization, overall team performance must be maintained at a high level.

CHAPTER TEN

MENTORING

One of the main functions for a leader in academic medicine is to ensure a steady inflow of young physicians and scientists into medicine. The profession cannot afford to have anything go awry with this talent pipeline. The greatness of our healthcare system in the United States is, for the most part, a result of the research engine in the biomedical sciences that has developed over the last century. Physicians and scientists are trained in medical schools of our AHCs and the research largely financed by the government through the National Institutes of Health. Research scientists working in concert with scientists at the National Institutes of Health, in the laboratories of the pharmaceutical and biotech companies, and at research institutes throughout the United States have produced an extraordinary wealth of new medical knowledge leading to a better understanding of human disease and remarkable advances in improving the diagnosis and treatment of many diseases. The beneficiaries are the American people and patients around the world. With each passing year, the research pipeline of scientists needs to be constantly replenished to keep the quality and numbers of scientists at an optimal level.

I have said on several occasions in earlier chapters in this book that it is not easy for a young medical student or postgraduate trainee (intern, resident or fellow) to figure out how best to train for a position in academic medicine in our system. Everyone entering the profession who wants to pursue the traditional career of teaching, research, and patient care needs advice from knowledgeable, accomplished and successful mentors. Most of the physicians and future scientists emanating from our medical schools find themselves, at the conclusion of medical school, deeply in debt because of high tuitions and the ancillary costs of attending medical school, such as room and board. The road they travel to attain career goals requires patience and sacrifice to train for their chosen field of expertise, acquire the necessary tools and achieve faculty status. Students must have a first-rate mentor or mentors because there are many questions that must be answered and advice tendered to the mentee.

I have been blessed in my career with a series of mentors from medical school through postgraduate training and throughout my time of active service at Miami, Pittsburgh and UCLA. Some of these mentors were not at my institutions but were national figures whom I met in the course of national meetings in which I presented my research findings. All of my mentors were with me every step of the way, providing the needed advice and recommendations for success that are so important.

They were truly extraordinary people and I would like to provide a brief picture about what these physicians and scientists were like as mentors, starting with my medical school. The relationship with my mentors over the years defined a near-perfect mentor-mentee interaction.

Seton Hall College of Medicine

In Chapter One I provided a concise overview of my early life and my beginning career in medical school. As a medical student at the Seton Hall College of Medicine, I knew from the very beginning that I wanted to do something special with my doctorate degree in medicine. I loved my time in medical school and the challenge of learning new medical material every hour of every day. My scholastic record was superb and I finished second in my class. During my four years of medical school, many of the professors at Seton Hall College of Medicine recognized something in my performance that they believed marked me with the potential to have an outstanding career in academics.

My earliest mentor in medical school was the woman I would eventually marry, Dr. Barbara Levey, who attended the State University of New York Upstate Medical University in Syracuse, New York. She was an inspiration to me: her academic excellence, integrity, confidence in me and willingness to share with me her views and a life together working hard to meet the challenges presented by a career in academic medicine for a two medical career family.

During my third year, which was the beginning of the clinical experience a student had in medical school, the chairman of medicine, the late Harold Jeghers, MD, identified me for a career in academics. He was an extraordinary teacher and one of the great clinicians of his time. Although today he would be classified as a clinician/teacher, he recognized the importance of biomedical research to have a truly great, full service Academic Health Center. His importance to me as a mentor was that he demonstrated the excitement of clinical medicine; he took me on some of his trips in which he was invited by physicians in local hospitals in the New York/New Jersey area who requested that he see patients of theirs because of his superb consultative abilities. They would present the cases; he would offer his diagnostic assessment and the needed therapeutic interventions. You can imagine the impression Dr. Jeghers had on me when he, one of the great physicians of his time, introduced me to his audience and patients. His impact was further strengthened by his towering height of 6'4", the fact that he drove a small sports car, wore a beret and I was the impressionable, third year medical student sitting beside him (height 5'6"). It was not only a first rate intellectual experience, but I would mull over in my mind the significance that he would think highly enough of me to make many of his consultative rounds part of my monthly educational activities. It was not surprising that later on I identified strongly with becoming a chairman of medicine. To this day, his picture hangs on my wall in my office suitably inscribed. In later life, he visited Barbara and me as frequently as he could, stayed at our home and regaled us with stories of the old days at Boston University and Georgetown.

Another mentor also appeared in the middle of my third year. I had read an article in a review journal on an entity called Tietze's syndrome. The report described a disease with costo-chondral (rib junction) pain, swelling and tenderness and the diagnosis was frequently confused with angina pectoris. This disease was rarely mentioned in the medical literature. Several months later, I made the diagnosis of Tietze's syndrome in one of my clinic patients and decided to write this up for the rheumatologic medical literature. The late Dr. John Calabro, professor and chief of the Division of Rheumatology, decided he would help me because after reading my initial draft, which I asked him to read, he felt I needed to learn writing skills. We worked together on the paper; I wrote and he rewrote all the while guiding me so that writing became a learning experience. The article was published in *Arthritis and Rheumatism*, an important journal in the field.

About a year later, I diagnosed the first case of Polymyalgia Rheumatica in the United States. The disease is characterized by aching in all the large joints, shoulder, hips, knees, without discernable damage to the joint. The only laboratory test, as a clue to the diagnosis, was an extremely high sedimentation rate. I made the diagnosis and treated the patient with steroids for several days; after we stopped the steroids, she was symptom free. After discharge, I told Dr. Calabro I wanted to write this up for *Arthritis and Rheumatism* and again we worked together on the article. After writing two scientific articles, I began writing articles for the medical literature. I will always be grateful to him for what he did for me; teaching me about medical writing and spending hours with me despite his busy schedule.

Another mentor, the late Dr. Carroll Leevy, Chief of the Division of Hepatology, provided key advice and friendship over the next thirty years and made certain that I was nominated to all the important societies.

During my senior year of medical school, I was approached by Dr. Philip Henneman, professor and Chief of the Division of Endocrinology, at Seton Hall. Dr. Henneman was a disciple of Dr. Fuller Albright generally acknowledged to be one the very best, if not the very best, endocrinologist of the 20th century. Dr. Henneman explained to me that medicine was changing. The infusion of dollars into the NIH and the explosion of medical knowledge that was beginning to occur because of an expanded research effort in the United States after

World War II indicated to him that to be a successful academician, you had to be a credible research scientist. Because I had no experience in this area, he recommended that I apply to the Harvard Medical School for a postdoctoral research fellowship in biological chemistry. I thought about this suggestion, discussed it with my wife and took a chance on doing something radically new. I applied for the fellowship and was accepted.

The thought of interrupting my residency and being located in a department at Harvard where everyone was a PhD (although the one person with an MD/PhD would be my preceptor) was intimidating, and I was scared. The experience I had with Dr. Joseph Alpers, Professor of Biological Chemistry, was amazing. I learned what Dr. Henneman told me I would, i.e., the rudiments of scientific research; and it enabled me in future years to be the credible research scientist that he said was necessary. After completing my two year fellowship, I finished my clinical training at Massachusetts General Hospital and was then off to the National Institutes of Health for four years where I was a member of the United States Public Health Service and a clinical associate at the National Institutes of Health. I learned much from the scientists at the National Institutes of Health; in particular, Dr. Ira Pastan, who was my laboratory chief for my first two years at NIH, and Dr. Gopal Krishna. After finishing four years, the last two of which were in the cardiology branch of the National Institutes of Health, my research career was going full steam.

After my tenure at the National Institutes of Health, I became a faculty member at the University of Miami School of Medicine and later, when I left Miami to become chairman of medicine at the University of Pittsburgh, I met four of the most extraordinary individuals who served as my mentors in the later years of my career. Dr. David Kipnis, former chairman of the Department of Medicine at the Washington University School of Medicine, Dr. Eugene Braunwald, former chairman of the Department of Medicine at the Brigham and Women's Hospital and Harvard Medical School, the late Dr. Robert Petersdorf, former president of the Association of American Medical Colleges and the late Dr. Thomas Detre, former president of the Medical and Healthcare Division of the University of Pittsburgh, provided the most extraordinary mentoring possible. All of these senior scientists, clinicians, administrators and leaders of American medicine once again saw something in me which made me special. They guided me through some of the more difficult areas for any young physician scientist embarking on his first management job as chair of medicine. They were always available for me by phone, and Drs. Kipnis, Braunwald and Petersdorf served as an external board of advisors committee for the department of medicine at the University of Pittsburgh. Dr. Detre was very influential by recommending me and strongly supporting my candidacy for the position at UCLA as dean of the David Geffen School of Medicine and vice chancellor of Medical Sciences. Would that everyone have mentoring such as I received in my career.

With a profound need for mentoring, it is an important role for the leader(s) at our medical institutions. First, the leader can ensure that he or she personally mentors members on his or her team, many of whom will benefit from his or her experiences in professional life.

Second, medicine, especially academic medicine, remains a somewhat hierarchical profession. There are many hurdles to overcome to progress from medical student to full professorship. Most medical students, residents or assistant professors must deal with medical school debt from rising tuitions and the time it takes to fully train in a specialty/subspecialty and the economic sacrifice of entering academic medicine as a career. In addition, the medical profession in general and particularly academic medicine can be challenging for trainees and younger faculty members when they are confronted with navigating and understanding the politics of medicine. Helping trainees and junior faculty is a must for the leader who can provide the mentoring structure. That structure and the leader needs to create an environment that is friendlier to generating the future leaders of the profession in all spheres of interest whether it be research, patient care, teaching or combinations thereof.

The leader must stress that everyone in the organization has an obligation to give back, including the leader. Most successful leaders in American medicine have been the beneficiaries of the type of mentoring described in this chapter that I received. Mentoring can occur at all levels of the AHC. Medical students can mentor other medical students. Senior housestaff can mentor junior housestaff; senior faculty can and should mentor medical students and housestaff, and the same holds for the entire organization.

Mentors must be available to answer questions that include: how to combine research, patient care and teaching into a successful career; how much research training is required to be successful researcher; who is more able to attract extramural funds on a long-term basis; where to receive your training; what are the necessary qualifications for promotion; the necessity of acquiring a second advanced degree, such as PhD, MPH, MBA, or Master of Science, in order to be a more credible scientist. My mentors answered all these questions and directed me to the pathways through which an academician was required to take. I had no doubt of what was ahead of me because of the mentoring they provided.

I am confident that the leadership of academic medicine will recognize the important need for mentoring, to make mentoring part of the culture of the medical profession, thereby protecting our excellence as health care providers and the fragile ecosystems of quality patient care, and basic and clinical research. I hope that this book will play a role in mentoring the future leaders of academia because the skill set is in many ways complementary to the skill set to be a first-rate physician scientist, clinician educator or clinician teacher. I hope that this book and others like it will serve as the foundation for courses in leadership. Mentoring will be brought to a new level.

CHAPTER ELEVEN

GOVERNANCE BOARDS

There are many types of governance boards: Those that oversee for-profit businesses (some of which are publicly traded on the stock market, some are privately owned); some are not-for-profit, for example, private universities and some are public universities. The issues concerning these various boards and others not mentioned are very diverse. For example, the governing board of a major company traded on the stock market is concerned with stock price, profitability, integrity, all types of financial issues, product lines, mergers and acquisitions, and a host of issues that include not only domestic but international markets. The University of California Board of Regents, under whom I worked, also deal with complex financial issues and the integrity of its organization. However, the Board of Regents, and other boards like it in the university world has responsibilities to the public, the student body and faculty; issues of rising tuition; state budgets; environment for students; quality of the teachers; faculty satisfaction; facilities for teaching, including lecture halls and libraries, dormitories, the Academic Health Centers, and professional schools; parents of students; alumni; the K-12 public education system and diversity. For the reader not familiar with the University of California Academic Health Centers, there are currently five: University of California San Francisco, University of California Davis, University of California Los Angeles, University of California Irvine and University of California San Diego. A sixth, University of California Riverside, is hoping to admit its first class for the 2012–2013 academic school year.

The common denominator for any type of governance board is that it has ultimate responsibility for hiring the leader, performance of the organization, evaluation of the leader and removal of the leader, if necessary. Therefore, one of the important responsibilities for any leader in academia or business is developing a positive and productive relationship with the governance board of the institution or organization. You report to the board; they approved of you being hired; and this is a critical relationship that needs to be constantly and carefully nurtured. The leader must recognize that board members need to be treated with the utmost respect and kept well informed about problems and opportunities. Just as you expect "no surprises" from your direct reports, the leader should not surprise the board.

As previously mentioned, one of the leader's most important responsibilities is to clearly enunciate and describe the vision for moving the institution or business forward. At a very early stage in a newly-appointed leader's administration, he or she will be required to present a "State of the Organization." After the leader has had a chance to meet with all the key players and reorganize his or her team, there will be an opportunity to educate the board and teach them things they didn't know about the institution or business. It is imperative that they become acquainted with all of the strengths and weaknesses from your point of view, since "new eyes" generally produce a different view of the organization than they have become accustomed to. The goals you must and will outline for them over time must be presented in such a manner that they grasp the necessity of any action that is required; how you plan to accomplish it; how much it will cost to implement any new initiatives; and finally, sources of revenue, if any, that will be needed.

Assessment of personnel is another major responsibility of the leader since you generally have a period of time to change your direct reports in the organization either by reshuffling internally and/or by recruiting new people. Boards, in general, like stability as well as quality of personnel and need to have a comfort zone when personnel change. The individuals who are newly placed in a position, whether they are internal or external, need to be introduced to the Board, and must present their views of what functions and responsibilities they are fulfilling in your administration.

Any changes in mission, such as any possible mergers or acquisitions, usually require multiple sessions to present to the Board with an analysis of why the vision or mission change is necessary. A careful review of all of the ramifications for the organization, good or bad, and a cost analysis must be presented.

The Board must understand your internal organizational tree so they know who is whom in the pecking order. They must have the comfort of having a succession plan for your replacement in the event of a sudden departure or incapacitation of you or top direct reports. They must have supreme confidence in the financial management and the highest respect for the chief financial officer and your role in fiscal management. The Board must also be confident in your integrity, honesty and ethical approach to the issues, as well as your ability to keep the organization in the black financially. You have to earn their respect over time and achieve their highest confidence level by the way you manage the issues including steering the ship through any crisis.

The leader must develop a personal relationship with every member of the Board, they must get to know you as a person and, hopefully, they will get to know your family. These are important confidence builders. Contact with each and every board member also permits you to know them better: their personality, character and how they view the organization. If this is a board for an AHC and a board member asks you to help with a medical issue for them, their family, friends or acquaintances, you must do so promptly. There is no better education for the board member than to experience healthcare at "their" hospital or clinic with one of the institutional physicians and staff, such as nurses. These positive interactions are additional confidence builders. Finally, you must always keep in mind that the board members are dedicated, hard working and concerned about serving in the public interest. They don't *need* more work in their busy lives, but choose to serve voluntarily. This makes them very special people indeed.

The functions just described for interactions with the Board will, in many instances, turn out to be pivotal in the success or failure of a leader's administration of the institution or organization. If the Board does not understand what you are doing and why, it is unlikely that you will garner the support that is necessary for success as a leader.

CHAPTER TWELVE

ADVICE FOR SEARCH COMMITTEES

When I was asked to interview for the position of dean of the UCLA School of Medicine and provost for Medical Sciences, I discussed with the chairperson of the search committee, Dr. Gary Tischler, the reasons that motivated the governance change of UCLA's Academic Health Center. Dr. Tischler told me that the University had decided that there would be one leader of UCLA's Academic Health Center to whom all others in the medical organization would report, including the hospital director. In the prior governance structure, the hospital director reported to the chancellor, whereas the dean of the medical school reported to the executive vice chancellor. Chancellor Charles Young and Executive Vice Chancellor Andrea Rich implemented this change in governance because of the deep concerns they had about a growing sense of conflict within the medical area. The medical school and the hospital were not working together in the requisite cooperative and collegial manner that is necessary to fulfill the missions of both units. Discord at the top was impeding the medical school's ability to achieve its full academic potential. Furthermore, the clinical mission also needed full cooperation of the parties to be successful in the era of managed care that was challenging the delivery of healthcare in California. Dr. Tischler also told me that in order to smooth the transition to the new governance paradigm, Dr. Andrea Rich had been serving in the capacity of provost until the new provost/dean was in place.

I arrived at UCLA for my first interview the Friday before the Northridge Earthquake in January 1994. The search committee impressed me in several ways. Although it was rather large, being comprised of sixteen people, the committee was composed of an interesting and heterogeneous mix of business people and campus leaders including the deans of the School of Law, School of Management and School of Dentistry. The level of questioning was superior to any I had encountered in my interviews for medical deanships over the previous seven or eight years. The first interview at UCLA was about an hour and a half to two hours in length; I was challenged with questions regarding my management style, especially by the business people. One question I remember quite clearly was how I made decisions in a large, complex organization; another was how I would communicate with faculty and staff; still others were directed at my personal values.

As Candidate Levey, I drew a number of conclusions. One, this committee was serious about their task; two, they knew what they were doing and asked the right questions; three, the business people added greatly to this committee asking relevant and challenging questions; and four, they appreciated the risks inherent in the new governance structure and its importance to the future of UCLA's Medical Sciences. I had two additional interviews over the ensuing four months which served to solidify the opinions I developed during and after the first interview.

The point I am trying to make is that the profession of medicine and the governance of large AHCs has become highly complex; these jobs require a leader to have a variety of career experiences and to possess people skills (see Chapter Three; Personal Value Scale) including: honesty, integrity, high ethical values, work ethic, keeping promises that are made, communication, being respectful and having a sense of humor. I later learned that the search committee was impressed with the variety of positions I had held in my professional career which made for a very comprehensive experience. In particular, they viewed as a strong positive my experiences at Merck. One person told me several years later that my time at Merck was decisive for my candidacy. This came as a mild surprise since several of my friends in academia were dismayed at my leaving academia for the world of the big pharmaceutical companies.

Finally, the main conclusion is that the chancellor, the executive vice chancellor and the search committee clearly and appropriately recognized the need for a different and more rigorous search process because the institutional stakes were so high. Failure in selection could have resulted in irreparable damage to UCLA's medical school and hospital.

With this backdrop of my experience with the search committee at UCLA, what advice can I offer to search committees, boards of trustees and to the search firms that work with universities and businesses to recruit the future leaders of medical institutions or businesses? First, and perhaps most important, is a recognition that times are changing dramatically in the field of medicine and perhaps even for corporations and small businesses who are facing the prospects of increasing governmental regulation. Recent developments in research and health-care reform are revolutionary in scope and it is hard to predict what will be the final outcome on the field of medicine and all aspects of the health and welfare of Americans. Universities, businesses and their search committees and the search firms they hire will be seeking this next generation of leaders at a time of great change and great opportunities. Making mistakes in selection will be costly and the selection process must be efficient, effective, and thorough, and conducted with everyone having knowledge of the required skill set.

In medicine we have entered another golden age of science with the emergence of (genetics) as a likely formidable tool which will permit the recognition of a disease or a patient's susceptibility to a disease even before the disease is clinically manifest. Preventive measures should come to the forefront as a major consequence of genetic medicine. Genetic medicine should also be a major tool for "curing" a disease before it happens by preventing it's ever happening. Preventive medicine hopefully will emerge as the vehicle for driving down healthcare expenditures because it is far cheaper to prevent the disease from occurring than it is to have the disease attain recognition as a clinical entity producing signs and symptoms in the patient. The simple intervention of smoking cessation in genetically susceptible individuals is certainly a more efficient and effective way to decrease the number of cases of lung cancer, kidney cancer, bladder cancer, oral cancers including tongue and throat, emphysema and bronchitis, to name a few. Ultimately, it is hoped that gene therapy will reach a technological breakthrough permitting physician scientists to replace missing or defective genes and, hopefully, be decisive in eliminating diseases such hemophilia, sickle cell anemia and hemochromatosis.

The era of stem cell medicine as a tool to provide insight into understanding the mechanisms of disease is rapidly approaching fruition. This newly developing field may serve to provide replacement pancreatic beta cells to patients with type 1 and some forms of type 2 diabetes mellitus. Other avenues of stem cell research may promote regeneration of neural tissue for those with spinal cord injuries. The ability to use one's own cells to regenerate organs for transplantation could become a reality in the next several decades, eliminating the tragedy of long waiting lines for organs and enable the recipients to resume normal lives sooner.

The era of targeted therapies for cancer has begun and proven decisive in treating several forms of cancer, for example, chronic myelogenous leukemia (gleevec) and certain types of breast cancer (herceptin). A great deal of effort is being expended based on the early success of targeted therapy. These scientific initiatives in genetic medicine, the application of stem cells to the understanding, diagnosis, and treatment of human disease and the utilization of targeted therapies has the potential to reverse and radically decrease by many billions of dollars the expenditure for healthcare, and to invigorate the economy.

Healthcare reform legislation recently passed by Congress will over time change our healthcare system as we know it. Many people do not understand this legislation, many people may not want this legislation to reach fruition and others are passionate about the legislation as providing much needed reform. Whoever is right about the legislation, there is no going back. The major thrust of this legislation focuses on the structure of the healthcare system in the United States. Methods of reimbursement, healthcare available through work benefits, and consideration of rationing of care, including the availability of advanced technology and treatment to patients will be at the forefront of change. Physicians, hospitals, insurance companies, pharmaceutical and biotech companies, small and large businesses and their work-force that heretofore received health benefits from their employers will have to navigate through all this, and it will be a formidable challenge for all of us.

It is against this backdrop that the future leaders of American medicine and American businesses will be recruited; they will be thrust into the middle of great change in society and will face unprecedented challenges. Whether the leader is a university president, the head of the university's AHC, a dean, a vice chancellor, a department chair or division chief, the leaders being recruited will need to be rigorously screened for skill sets and traits they *must* possess, which historically most search committees and search firms have not utilized in their attempts to find the best people to serve as leaders. Universities, businesses, boards of trustees, search committees and search firms will have to develop prototypes for these leadership positions. In my mind, as the 21st century evolves, leaders will need a broad range of skills and must be prepared to handle challenges in research, clinical medicine, education, hospitals, finances, team building, and possess the personal values already reviewed in Chapter Three. The times are too perilous to have leaders serve only a short tenure. Generally speaking, a ten to fifteen year tenure for the leader to learn about the challenges, effect necessary changes and implement thoughtful new initiatives is about the right length of time.

CHAPTER THIRTEEN

CRISIS MANAGEMENT

Dr. Thomas Rosenthal and Ms. Dale Tate have played a key role in Crisis Management during my tenure at UCLA and continue in that role today. At my request, they organized the Crisis Management Team which included themselves and our outside counsels Messrs. Louis M. Marlin and Stanley Saltzman, who helped with strategy and execution. In addition, Dr. Rosenthal and Ms. Tate defined the role for the leader and maintained a detailed record of the facts regarding the several crises we experienced during my fifteen years at UCLA. They are uniquely qualified to lead our crisis management efforts; Dr. Rosenthal is chief medical officer of the Ronald Reagan UCLA Medical Center and associate vice chancellor and Ms. Tate is executive director of Health Sciences Communication and Government Relations. Therefore, I asked them to undertake the task of writing this chapter. My contribution was editing the text to try to provide a degree of literary continuity and homogeneity. I hope we have succeeded; this chapter is an important part of any text dealing with leadership.

Inevitability

For many years, physicians were considered "gods" by most lay people — and quite a few saw themselves that way. But medicine is as much an art as a science, and doctors are human, with all the same frailties and vulnerabilities as any other man or woman. With increasing scrutiny by the outside world — the media, government, public interest groups—issues like medical errors, conflicts-of-interest and patient privacy breaches are now very much in the public eye. Given the complexity of our institutions and what we do, it is inevitable that even the finest academic health centers will have a "crisis" from time to time. How the institution handles these crisis situations, however, is a true measure of leadership.

The instinctive reaction when something goes wrong is to circle the wagons and do everything possible to contain information. That may have worked in the 20th century, but in the day of the 24 hour news cycle, the Internet, social media, and most of all, a society that values transparency, that approach can't, and frankly shouldn't, work. Those of us in academic medicine have a responsibility to all of our constituencies — our students, patients, faculty, staff, university administrators, and donors — to be honest and forthcoming. And if we work at public institutions, we are obligated to advise the public when things go wrong, just as we put out press releases when we do something remarkable. Some of the most difficult battles a leader may face in crisis situations will pit them against those who want to keep those wagons in place. Lawyers, by the nature of the work they do, campus administrators and those directly involved in the crisis may argue to keep information about the event(s) closely contained. But that is the wrong path for two reasons (a) it won't work and (b) the public has a right to know.

Knowledge is Power

Once a leader knows about a crisis situation, the first thing she or he must do is gather all the relevant facts. In difficult situations, every bit of information must be gathered; information about the individuals involved including personnel records, background checks, résumés and job applications; a detailed timeline of what happened; local, state and federal laws and regulations that may have been violated; as well as internal campus and medical rules and regulations; and determining who in the institution had knowledge of the event. All of this information is critical to developing a strategy for how to respond.

Having a solid, trusted team is necessary for just about everything you do as the leader of an academic health center, but it is probably most important in times of crisis. From that solid, trusted team, a leader can begin creating a rapid response group that will include senior legal, communications, and administrative personnel. These are the people that will do the heavy lifting — do the detailed background work, develop messaging, and coordinate with other offices and stakeholders, on campus and off. Needless to say, it is essential that this team is comprised of people the leader not only trusts, but whose professional abilities are respected.

Even in the frantic atmosphere of a crisis, preparation and training are key to getting through the situation. Here is where experienced, skilled professional staffers are critical. Once all the relevant information is gathered, it is the rapid response group that will determine a plan of action, which must be approved. They will help decide who will be the spokesperson, what are the key message points, develop all the communications materials (speeches, press releases, fact sheets, letters, etc.) and if time permits, media training.

Crises tend to take on a life of their own. So the leader must remain flexible, adjusting as new information comes to light and as unexpected players become involved. The leader will be getting advice from all corners, but this is when trust in the team comes into play. If the leader has a strategy that is reflective of the basic principles of honesty and transparency, and the appropriate people to carry out that strategy, one can weather the storm.

Managing today's 24/7 media environment is not easy, but web-based communications, such as social media, actually can help in crisis situations since one does not have to rely upon mainstream media to tell the story. But the story must contain the three A's of crisis management:

- Acknowledge

- Apologize

- Act

If one has proof that the crisis situation is real, one must be forthright and acknowledge the problem. The truth will always come out; if one takes responsibility for it, then one has a much better chance to help control how people perceive the problem. In the past, lawyers have been very reluctant for clients to say "I'm sorry." But in a situation where the institution(s) or its employee(s) are clearly at fault, it's imperative to thoughtfully and sincerely express regret and apologize. It will not placate everyone impacted by the crisis, but it will go a long way toward smoothing the waters. Finally, once the "mea culpa" has been made, one has to explain what they're going to do to ensure that a similar problem doesn't happen again. It's not enough to say you're sorry; one has to lay out concrete steps — a plan of action, both short and long-term — to assure the public.

On the other hand, if there is a difficult situation, but no one at the institution has made an error, no one has violated any law, but events that have taken place will be perceived negatively by the public, one must work with the team to present all the facts and be prepared to take some hits from the external world. Situations like the unpredicted death of a young child, or providing organ transplants to prisoners or foreign nationals, are examples of this conundrum. The institution has done absolutely nothing medically, ethically, or legally wrong, yet the media may portray it and the public may perceive it negatively. In these situations, all one can do is present the facts and attempt to educate the public about difficult and complex medical issues.

CASE STUDY

Probably the best way to illustrate how to manage a crisis is to take a concrete example from my own experience at UCLA.

You may remember that in March 2004, during an internal investigation, the UCLA School of Medicine uncovered evidence that the director of the Willed Body Program, aided and abetted by an outside middleman, allegedly set up a side business selling bodies and body parts.

Crises come in all shapes and sizes. But when you have one that combines a major, well-respected institution, dead bodies and body parts, doctors and alleged criminals, there is little question that it's going to be huge. UCLA's willed body story was on the front pages of newspapers coast-to-coast, network news shows, and publications from highly respected academic journals to super-market tabloids — even Oprah called for interviews. But before getting to how we handled the crisis, I'd like to take a minute to give you a little background on UCLA's Willed Body Program to help put all of this in context.

In 1950, the year before the UCLA School of Medicine admitted its first class, the chair of anatomy, Dr. Horace Magoun, came up with the idea for a Willed Body Program and lobbied the California legislature to enact the Anatomical Gift Act, which authorized a person to will his or her body to a medical institution. It was the first such program in the country, and the first such law, although most other states have similar laws now in effect.

Prior to the scandal, an average of 175 people donated their bodies to UCLA each year. Virtually every department of the UCLA Center for Health Sciences depends on human cadavers to develop new, lifesaving procedures and facilitate the training of surgeons and, of course, to teach medical students the basics of human anatomy.

Unfortunately, the problems that were discovered in 2004 were not the first to beset UCLA's Willed Body Program. In the early 1990s, issues were raised about the disposal of the ashes of those who had donated their bodies to the program. There were accusations that cremated remains were mixed with scalpels and other material when they were disposed of at sea. Several class action suits were brought against UCLA — cases that were just about to be resolved in UCLA's favor — when this new scandal broke. And, by the way, the man who was hired in the early '90s to clean up our program and ensure that it was a model for willed body programs nation-wide, was the UCLA employee arrested in 2004, and subsequently found guilty.

The core facts are that the Willed Body Program director received personal payments for selling body parts to an outside broker in violation of UCLA Policy and Law. The thefts were uncovered by an internal audit team. When my office was notified, I put together a small team (noted in the introduction to this chapter on crisis management) to help me determine the facts and to prepare for the inevitable media coverage.

Our communications staff had made all the preparations necessary for a press conference on Monday and drafted a press release, a statement that was to be read by Dr. J. Thomas Rosenthal, who had done media training as had the chief of the UCLA Police Department. In fact, the training went beyond the typical rehearsing of message points. Extended "murder board" sessions were held, where they went through the "what ifs" a reporter asks this question, does that response make sense, does it stand up. Messages were tested not only for their accuracy, but for their believability, whether they conveyed the right tone and the sense of seriousness the situation demanded.

Our strategy for making the public announcement was contingent upon the police arresting the individuals involved in the sale of the body parts. We had our fingers crossed the entire week before the planned press conference that no one would leak the story. Somehow, we managed to keep the story under wraps for one whole week, but on Friday afternoon, March 5th, a *Los Angeles Times* reporter called our media relations office asking for a response to information he had received from "highly placed sources" at UCLA that someone was selling bodies and body parts from our Willed Body Program.

During the days between when we first learned of the investigation and that phone call from the *Los Angeles Times*, we did an incredible amount of spade work. For starters, we drafted a holding statement that we had ready to send to the *LA Times* reporter immediately after he called. We had prepared a detailed media strategy, developed key message points, had several media training sessions for our designated spokespersons, put together a lengthy list of questions and answers we anticipated fielding, and made all the necessary arrangements for the press conference.

When the first story broke in the *LA Times* on Saturday morning, all hell broke loose. Our media relations office was inundated with press calls, local and national, but the prior week's preparation paid off. We had a prepared statement. We knew the message we wanted to convey in interviews, we knew what we could say, what we couldn't, and we had selected the best people to deliver those messages. A story like this takes on a life of its own, and you have to be adept at changing course, if required. For instance, we had initially planned on Dr. Rosenthal making the key statement at the press conference. But when it became clear how big the story was, I was convinced that I needed to deliver those remarks. And later that first week, when we learned that the court handling the earlier class action suits would probably shut down the Willed Body Program, our attorneys announced at the court hearing that we were voluntarily suspending operation of the program at the same time we were releasing a statement with that decision to the public.

It was about this same time that we brought in an outside public relations firm to verify that from an external relations perspective, we were handling the situation properly. They confirmed that we were on point. There are only two real reasons to hire outside public relations consultants: you don't trust your own people — not what a good leader would want; or you want to verify that you are doing things right.

I'd be the last person to say that we handled all this perfectly, seamlessly. The best you can do with a bad situation like this is try to not make it worse and mitigate the damage, but I believe we managed to do the following:

- First, we stepped up to the plate and admitted responsibility. We apologized to the families of those who had donated their bodies to the program and might have been victims of these crimes.
- Second, we pledged to cooperate fully with the authorities.
- Third, we made a commitment to correct our mistakes. We quickly named an outsider — former California Governor George Deukmejian — to undertake a thorough investigation of what went wrong and why. That initial investigation led to the naming

of a UC system-wide panel that, working together with a consultant, developed a wide-ranging set of reforms which were implemented at the five UC medical schools and became a national model for willed body programs.

But, in addition to taking care of the media, we had to address concerns we were sure would arise with several special interest groups, most relatively easy to contend with, the other, very difficult.

The first was our internal constituency; the medical school faculty and staff; the medical students; hospital physicians and staff; the greater campus community; alumni; and donors. To address these groups, we took a multi-pronged approach:

- The chancellor sent an e-mail message to all faculty and staff, which was also posted on the UCLA home page.
- I sent a personal e-mail message to all medical school faculty and staff, and all hospital personnel and medical students.
- I also did a lengthy question & answer piece on the Willed Body Program, the investigation, and our plan of action for our staff/faculty newsletter, which is published every other week.
- We provided ready access of all relevant materials to reporters from the student newspaper, the *Daily Bruin*, which is the student body's main news source.
- We worked with the alumni association so they would be prepared to respond to any questions, and helped the government

relations staff prepare background materials that were sent to all members of the Los Angeles delegation in Sacramento and Washington, DC.

- Finally, I called key donors to personally apprise them of what had happened and what steps we were taking to address the problem.

The much more difficult special interest group to address was the families. While those donating their bodies to the program were fully briefed about how their cadavers might be used before they signed all appropriate legal documents, there was nothing that required these individuals to go home and explain those details to his or her family. The only thing the families may have been told was that their mom or dad, husband or wife donated his or her body to UCLA. They might assume that it was going to be used by a medical student to learn gross anatomy, or a surgeon in training. But more than likely, they didn't know that the body might be divided up so that a cardiologist could do research on the heart, an orthopedic surgeon could practice a new technique on the knee, and our brain mapping center might slice the brain into thin sheets to record and catalog as part of our Brain Atlas initiative.

So when the *LA Times*, and others, ran stories about the middleman cutting up bodies in the hospital and spiriting the parts out during the dead of night, well, you can imagine that many of the families reacted with shock and dismay.

We tried to anticipate the fallout and took what now have become standard measures:

- We set up a website with basic information about the program and its status along with an e-mail address that individuals could use to ask questions.
- We also created a hotline for concerned individuals to call. The phones were answered by nurses, who recorded names and contact information and advised callers — most were family members — that we would get back to them as soon as we had any information. Every press release and statement included the website address and the hotline number, and the local media included them both in their coverage.

Unfortunately, because there was an ongoing police investigation, we did not have access to the Willed Body Program files. And we knew that it might take many months before we could determine which bodies had been handled properly and which might be part of the criminal investigation. In fact, we were told it was very likely there would be a number of bodies that we would never be able to definitively put into one category or the other.

After a month, we recognized we had to do something more for the families, but there were legal constraints. Days after the scandal hit the press, three new class action lawsuits were filed against UCLA. Each and every one of those family members was now a potential litigant. Our lawyers finally agreed to allow us to send letters to those family members who had contacted the hotline, since we were merely responding to their queries, not trying to influence them in any way. That letter took many days to finalize, with six attorneys, in addition to several doctors and campus administrators, vetting each word.

A senior hospital administrator was appointed the Willed Body Program liaison, a woman who directed our risk management office and was skilled at dealing with irate, emotional, and distraught people. By this time the number of calls had dwindled down to a dozen or so a week, but those who called were repeat callers, anxious, angry, and ones who needed special care.

After several weeks, the daily news stories ended, but the coverage continued for more than a year. Now every time there is an incident involving the sale of body parts, UCLA is usually mentioned. One of the criminals — not a UCLA employee — wrote a book entitled, *Willing Bodies… Inside the UCLA Willed Body Program.* We got a bit of coverage when the 200 plus page "Willed Body Report," which presented a detailed plan to reform all the University of California willed body programs, was presented to the University's Board of Regents. I was disappointed, but not surprised, that the subsequent stories did not focus on how the programs would all be standardized, the revamped reporting system that was being instituted, or the enhanced over-sight of the program.

UCLA was hit hard and heavy. I've been told that this was the worst scandal in the institution's history. It certainly was the most stressful time of my professional life, especially the 96 hours leading up to the press conference. Now that the trial has taken place, and the perpe-trators found guilty of grand theft, tax evasion and sentenced to prison terms, it is apparent that in fact, UCLA was also a victim of a crime. Yet, despite the Jay Leno jokes and salacious headlines, I really don't believe there has been any lasting damage to the institution. UCLA's David Geffen School of Medicine is still standing, doing what it does best, teaching and training a new generation of physicians, doing ground-breaking research and treating patients.

CHAPTER FOURTEEN

FUND-RAISING

From the interview stage to the earliest weeks of my tenure as the vice chancellor and dean, it was apparent that there was an urgency to focus on the development of a major fund-raising effort to provide capital for buildings, programs, endowed chairs and unrestricted endowment. California was in the midst of a serious recession and much work needed to be done to reinvigorate the medical enterprise. I began to initiate a strategy for fund-raising. At the same time, however, I was not absolutely confident I could succeed because as a faculty member at the University of Miami School of Medicine, it was not part of my job description. However, I did garner experience in fund-raising at the University of Pittsburgh School of Medicine. The modest exposure I had at Pitt came in the first two years of my tenure when I had two successful forays into the world of philanthropy. One of my goals was to begin an industrial and occupational medicine program but the Department of Medicine was lacking the necessary startup funds, of approximately $300,000. I was able to secure an introduction and meeting with David Roderick who at that time was the chief executive officer and chairman of United States Steel. We met on two occasions in his office in downtown Pittsburgh and I explained my reasons for the program and the request. I stressed that I believed our community, the steel industry and medical school should develop a first class program in occupational and industrial healthcare. Mr. Roderick was somewhat hesitant at first because, as he pointed out to me, the University of Pittsburgh was a state related institution that received taxpayer support and therefore was already receiving financial support, albeit indirectly, from US Steel and its employees. I explained that although we were state related, we received an inadequate amount of money compared to what we needed to operate a first-class department and academic health center. To his great credit, Mr. Roderick believed our discussion about helping the workers was critical and he agreed with my goals and objectives. He agreed to provide the entire sum of $300,000 for this program. I was thrilled and it was my first successful undertaking in fund-raising. The second effort was my attempt to initiate the first program in geriatrics in western Pennsylvania. This was one of my highest priorities because of the large number of people in western Pennsylvania who were over the age of 65. It was imperative therefore to initiate this program and make the Department of

Medicine more relevant in the area of healthcare specialized for the elderly. I was introduced to the chief executive officer of the Benedum Foundation in West Virginia, Paul Jenkins, who was fortuitously looking to invest in just such a program. We spoke on several occasions and finalized a $1,000,000 gift to start the Geriatric Program. These two gifts were a tremendous boon to the department and in those days a substantial sum of money. My career as a fund-raiser ended temporarily because a senior university official in the health sciences complained to the chancellor that he did not want department chairs raising money as it might position the departments in conflict with his priorities for philanthropy. I understood and did not seek any further opportunities to raise money for our department. However, I learned three basic principles from my brief foray into fund-raising at the University of Pittsburgh. These three principles are discussed below and are the first three of eight principles listed, and referred to as Levey's Principles for Fund-Raising.

Principle One: You need respected people in the community introducing you to the people of influence and affluence in the community.

I could not have made the connections with Messrs. Roderick and Jenkins without the introductions by an important figure at Pitt and the greater Pittsburgh area, Edison Montgomery, who was very effective in that role. Los Angeles, a much larger community and more affluent than Pittsburgh, posed a problem by having infinitely greater competition for philanthropic gifts. I was in the big leagues in Los Angeles and I needed some special champions, especially in the entertainment world in addition to the business world. In my first year in Los Angeles, in fact in my first meeting the day after I accepted the job, I was introduced to Michael Ovitz, the highly successful and powerful chairman of the Creative Artists Agency. Over time he introduced me to a who's who of the Los Angeles and Hollywood community. The second person to help me make connections was the director of development at the medical school, Mr. Michael Eicher. Eicher introduced me to Leslie and Susan Gonda in the second month after I started my job at UCLA. I was re-introduced to the Gonda's by our chair of urology, Dr. Jean deKernion, who already had developed a relationship with the family, but offered to help me in any way he could to help strengthen the Gonda's commitment to the institution. Both of their introductions led to my relationship with the Gonda's that culminated in April 1995 with the largest gift (at the time) in UCLA's history of $45,000,000 for building the Gonda (Goldschmied) Neuroscience and Genetics Research Center. This building enabled our school of medicine to provide the research space to begin a new Department of Human Genetics and to bring much needed changes to the Brain Research Institute and the entire neuroscience community at UCLA.

It helped that plans were already on the drawing board for a building designed by Robert Venturi that was part of our broader scheme of reinvigorating the neurosciences. The first meeting with the Gondas was key to everything that subsequently happened. They liked me and my plans for the School of Medicine, but they loved my wife Barbara, so as a team, she and I built the relationship with the Gondas that was so necessary to encourage them to invest in UCLA. The Gonda (Goldschmied) Neuroscience and Genetics Research Center has been an amazing success and ultimately the donors were so pleased it led to a series of other donations over the years that included the Gonda (Goldschmied) Vascular Center, the Gonda (Goldschmied) Diabetes Center, the Gonda/UCLA Robotic Surgery Center and the Gonda (Goldschmied) Cardiovascular Floor of our new Ronald Reagan UCLA Medical Center. After the fund-raising success in my first year with the Gonda family, I knew I could fund-raise and I was confident we would be successful in this arena. It was also important for our development office and faculty to know that fund-raising was possible and it could greatly impact our university and in particular the medical enterprise. My determination and confidence soared.

Principle Two: Be thoroughly prepared when soliciting a donor.

Whether in Pittsburgh, Los Angeles or any city, it is important to recognize that before meeting with anyone you must prepare, down to the smallest details for the specific donation, not only why you want it but how much you estimate it will cost, and to put it into context with the broader mission and goals of the medical enterprise. I knew the larger picture for both the school and hospital because of my job, which mandated a unified governance organization. When I finished relating my plans to the donors and/or their foundation directors, I wanted them to consider themselves partners in this effort to revitalize the medical school and hospital. In general it is important that the donor's foundation directors be informed since many donors depend on the foundation directors to provide a key perspective regarding the worthiness of the project or program.

You must provide a confidence building presentation demonstrating that you have the vision, enthusiasm and motivation to make things happen. People will not donate unless they perceive you to be a leader of a great enterprise that is not only viable but vibrant, and that we are all doing something that will make the university even greater.

Principle Three: Ask for what you need; don't try to guess what the donor will give.

In Pittsburgh I was fortunate enough that I asked and received what I needed for both the industrial and occupational medicine program and for the Benedum Geriatrics Center. Paul Jenkins, the CEO of the Benedum Foundation, knew what they wanted to donate and it was an amazing gift that made the recruitment of a top geriatrician possible and to establish the program quickly.

For the Gonda gift, arriving at the donation of $45,000,000 is an interesting story. In early April 1995, I received a phone call from Mr. Gonda. In the course of the conversation, he said he wanted to make a big gift to UCLA and wanted me to make an appointment to come to his office and discuss with him what we had available. I was able to get an appointment for about three weeks later, and at that meeting during the course of the conversation, I responded to his question about available opportunities by saying that my major goal was to endow and name the UCLA School of Medicine. We needed unrestricted funding in the form of an endowment to enable us to start new programs to recruit and retain the best faculty and to have adequate student scholarships to make our school competitive for the best and brightest students regardless of financial needs. I told him we were asking $250,000,000. He looked at me for what seemed like an eternity and said he hadn't planned on anything that big and in any event he wasn't interested in endowments. How I got up the nerve to ask for such a big donation I don't know, but I did, and although he said no to my large request, on the plus side, Mr. Gonda didn't throw me out of his office.

We discussed other options and then I told him about the building we had planned, designed by Robert Venturi, to house our neuroscience programs. I told him I wanted the building to be the home of our new Human Genetics Department and Brain Research Institute which was a key institute for the neuroscience faculty on the UCLA campus. The architectural plans had been completed about four years earlier and they allowed for an additional floor which would provide an ideal amount of laboratory space. Mr. Gonda expressed a strong preference for buildings over endowments. He asked what it would cost and I told him $45,000,000 which included the extra floor. I also mentioned that UCLA had already invested $10,000,000. He said he was very interested and wanted to have another meeting to review the plans. Several weeks later these plans were reviewed with Mr. Gonda and the donation was finalized about six weeks later when his lawyers and the University's lawyers completed the agreement. At that time, this was the largest single donation ever given to UCLA. I remain convinced to this day that the Gonda gift paved the way for the huge success of our capital campaign which began July 1, 1995 and concluded December 31, 2005.

Principle Four: Be patient, keep trying and never give up.

Requests for donations sometimes have to percolate and after you make a formal presentation you may not hear back from them for a while. Such was the case for the spectacular gift from David Geffen that resulted in naming and endowing the David Geffen School of Medicine at UCLA in 2002. In the year 2000, an appointment was arranged for me to meet with Mr. Andy Spahn, director of David Geffen's Foundation to make a formal presentation regarding the naming of the UCLA School of Medicine. The meeting occurred in the conference room next to my office. For the sixty minutes that was allotted, I discussed every facet of the school of medicine including reviews of our education, research, and clinical care programs. In addition, I discussed our mission and the vision I had for the school of medicine and why this gift was so vitally important for the future of the school. That meeting went well; at the conclusion, I felt very good about it and that I had bonded in a special way with Mr. Spahn. No timetable was proposed or given for hearing about a decision. I had done my best; time would tell.

To fill in the gaps for completeness, over the previous six or seven years I had made about a half dozen or so proposals to individuals worth over $1,000,000,000 to name the School of Medicine. The asking price was $250,000,000; some donors said they were unable to make such a large donation and others I never heard back from regarding this subject. All I knew is that I had to keep trying, as it was worth the effort.

I didn't hear anything about the proposal to David Geffen until March 2002. Approximately 18 months after my meeting with Mr. Spahn, the call came through from the central development office on the UCLA campus and the message I received was that Mr. Geffen wanted to discuss the naming gift; I was to call his office and meet him for lunch at his home in Beverly Hills. The meeting was arranged for April 4, 2002, a date I took as a good sign since it was the birth date of my dad who died when I was a teenager. Naturally, the day couldn't come fast enough for me. As an aside, at the time of the meeting, I was asking $150,000,000 for the endowment as we had reduced the asking price after coming to the conclusion that $250,000,000 seemed to be too steep, and two schools had recently been named for much less. Cornell University Medical College was named for a gift of $100,000,000 by Joan and Sandy Weill and the University of Southern California School of Medicine by the Keck Foundation for a gift of $110,000,000.

At the lunch meeting, Mr. Geffen and I became acquainted since we had not met prior to this and we also discussed the various features of the School of Medicine. After about an hour and half, he said he'd received a request from another university to name their medical school as well. That prompted him to "dust off the Levey proposal" because he lived right here in Los Angeles and if he was going to name a medical school, it would be more logical to do it close to home. When Mr. Geffen reviewed his reasons for this gift, he said he wanted to have a positive effect on healthcare in California; he thought the best way to do that was to train the finest medical students in California and to further medical research. He told me he was prepared to give $100,000,000 and that was a nonnegotiable offer. He asked if I would accept the gift and I responded affirmatively; I saw no obstacles and I was thrilled at the magnitude of this gift. I mentioned that his gift would represent the largest gift in the history of UCLA and the University of California. I also told him that I needed to review this proposal at a meeting with Chancellor Albert

Carnesale and secure his approval. As the meeting was breaking up, he asked me how I came to the conclusion that the naming opportunity was worth $150,000,000. I told him it was not rocket science and there was no mathematical formula. I considered UCLA to be one of the greatest medical schools in the United States and I believed that given its mission and the financial needs to fulfill that mission, that this endowment would provide the resources to keep UCLA at the forefront of biomedical research, patient care and education, and would ensure its future. He then followed that question up with another one: What was the largest gift ever made to a medical school? I told him I thought it was to Vanderbilt University in Tennessee, but told him I couldn't provide any specific details.

When I returned to UCLA, I quickly sought and received approval from the chancellor. In the ensuing four weeks, the lawyers for UCLA and for Mr. Geffen worked to finalize the terms of the gift. All of my requests were accepted: that the gift would be unrestricted, subject to the discretion of the dean and be a quasi-endowment. This would provide future deans with the ability to take from the corpus with the permission of the chancellor in order to invest in new programs and new recruitments. Within a month or so, the structure of the gift was completed and the chancellor and I signed the gift agreement. All that remained was for Mr. Geffen's signature.

Before that happened, I received a call stating that Mr. Geffen wanted to have another lunch meeting. I became slightly apprehensive; in being a lifelong sports fanatic, I knew the truth to the old maxim "it's never over until it's over." When the time arrived for the meeting, I was nervous but the meeting itself was quite relaxed and pleasant. Mr. Geffen said he checked on the largest gift ever made to a school of medicine and said to me as he held our agreement in his hand, "I think you will like this new version of our agreement." He handed me the document and when I read $200,000,000, I was both flabbergasted and ecstatic. He asked me to sign the approval for the terms of the gift, which I did; to this day I can remember the surprise, the excitement, the overwhelming feeling of accomplishment that the future of the new David Geffen School of Medicine at UCLA was secure. I asked him why he decided to double the size of the gift. He said he wanted to give the largest gift to a school of medicine because he wanted other people of similar or greater wealth to take his gift as a challenge to endow a medical school or endow their favorite institution.

After eight years of trying to fulfill this major goal of endowing the UCLA School of Medicine, it was done. Be patient, keep trying and never give up; principle number four!

Principle Five: Donors to AHCs expect the quid pro quo for their gifts: access to the best medical care.

At the very beginning of my tenure at UCLA, I learned from donors and from those individuals introducing me to potential donors that there exists an important quid pro quo for many of the donors, which is to facilitate access to first-class medical care at UCLA and even in some special instances to care at other medical institutions. Therefore I thought it prudent to formally organize a process in the dean's office to expedite the provision of access to medical care to donors, their families and friends who seek medical services.

Jane Cubicciotti was working in the dean's office when I arrived at UCLA in 1994; she had been serving as liaison to donors seeking medical care, although her role was not on the grand scale I envisioned in my planning for fund-raising. I appointed her assistant to the provost (later assistant to the vice chancellor) for Special Services and director, Division of Special Services. In her role as Director, Division of Special Services, she was fully responsible for continued development and expansion of the division, and developing and implementing policies as needed. Special Services operated on a 24/7 basis, responding swiftly to pages for emergencies, arranging medical referrals to physicians and facilities not only at UCLA, but nationwide and even worldwide. The division also responded to other requests from donors to provide medical assistance to family members and friends. Additionally, the division was responsive to requests from public officials, regents, other campus units and the chancellor as well as random calls for medical assistance that came directly to the dean/vice chancellor's office for the Medical Sciences.

The director of the division of Special Services and assistant to the vice chancellor reported directly to me, the vice chancellor for Medical Sciences. I felt a strong sense of obligation to our donors and others in the community and university and needed to be an active leader and participant in the Division of Special Services. I carried a pager 24/7 and the clinicians and hospital team knew of my level of involvement in the division and my commitment to the goals of the division. I made regular hospital visits and occasionally even went to the Emergency Department when one of the Special Services patients was receiving medical services. The director briefed me daily on new patients and follow-ups. Although I didn't realize it at the time, over the 15 years of my tenure, in actuality, what we created was one of the first concierge practices. I believed and continue to believe that a special bond is formed between those who experience the medical services of the Division of Special Services and the school of medicine, hospital system and university.

Having this service based in the office of the vice chancellor led to a sixth principle for fund-raising.

Principle Six: Don't compete with the faculty.

Providing access to medical care is not the same as providing the medical care. The physicians on the staff provide the care and many of them are looking to donors for some degree of philanthropic support

— for their research and/or clinical program or an endowed chair. They may develop resentment that the donors are being encouraged to focus on the institution and not the needs of the individual physician, scientist, department chair or division chief.

I had to be very sensitive to this issue and it was my policy to step aside for these individuals. Their proposal would come first. I felt that somehow it would work out to the benefit of all concerned and it was essential to have happy physician/scientists, stronger departments and divisions, as well as a stronger institution. To the best of my knowledge, it has always worked to the benefit of all. In the ten year capital campaign that ended on December 31, 2005, the total dollars raised for the medical sciences was $1,750,000,000, of which approximately $700,000,000 was directly attributable to the dean's office — including donor funding for five new research buildings of which three are named; approximately 110 new endowed chairs; the Geffen gift and a gift in excess of $150,000,000 to name the UCLA Medical Center for President Ronald Reagan.

Included in the $150,000,000 was a pivotal lead gift of $100,000,000 from Mr. Jerrold Perenchio, the chairman and CEO of Univision, a Spanish language communication network of TV and radio stations, and a distinguished alumnus of UCLA. Mr. Perenchio's extraordinary gift provided the decisive underpinning to build a seismically safe, technologically advanced 21st century hospital. Similar to Mr. Gonda,

Mr. Perenchio has also adopted other areas making personal donations to support physician/scientists, trainees and departments. On numerous occasions, Mr. Perenchio has demonstrated special loyalty and love both for his university and its hospital and medical school. This pattern of providing a pivotal major capital donation, followed by many faculty-oriented donations is further exemplified by Stewart and Lynda Resnick who named the Stewart and Lynda Resnick Neuropsychiatric Hospital at UCLA and have been major benefactors of the neurosciences. The Mattel Company, who named the Mattel Children's Hospital at UCLA, subsequently provided support over and above their capital gift to physician/scientists, research programs, training programs and endowed chairs. I feel quite fortunate to have circumvented any internal competition for donations which could impair relationships with faculty; one has to be on guard and never breech this line of etiquette.

Principle Seven: Philanthropy is a contact sport.

There are other expectations of the leader who is actively engaged in fund-raising. During my second year at UCLA, I was having a meeting with a wealthy potential donor — who several years later became a significant donor to the medical enterprise — and during the course of our conversation, he told me that "fund-raising is a contact sport." I had never heard that term used before and I asked him what he meant. He said that if you ask for philanthropic contributions to your area of interest, in this case it would be the UCLA medical enterprise, you are expected to reciprocate when solicited in turn by the donor for his or her charity of interest. I remarked that the levels of giving are on a different plane. He understood, but said it is the participation that matters, not necessarily the amount, which for me would be less than someone like himself could or would be expected to give.

My wife and I have always believed in giving back to the community in which we lived, however, we didn't know where this would lead in terms of our personal income as we looked at all the future fund-raising I had to do. As it turned out, we ultimately learned to tithe our income and felt that was appropriate for us. Whether or not this was a factor in my success as a fund-raiser, I can't say for sure. However, of one thing I am certain: my wife Barbara and I became a part of the Westside Los Angeles community, a very necessary feature of our life and position at UCLA and in Los Angeles. We attended many of the major events that occurred on the Westside of Los Angeles.

Principle Eight: Create a first-rate Office of Development.

Fund-raising is a complicated, high pressure and important fact of life for universities, and for the arts, disease advocacy groups, religious organizations, social services and political organizations to name a few. There is an expectation that these efforts be highly professional, ethical, honest and sensitive to the need to keep the expenses at a minimum. As a leader it is expected that you keep everyone on the development team familiar with the vision, the mission and goals of the institution as well as the goals of the various components, which have specific goals of their own. The leader must meet frequently with the director of development and his or her staff. The Development Office must be alert to identifying new prospects, nurturing those who have given in the past, planning events, and preparing many documents subsequent to the donation, which are scrutinized by lawyers on both sides. It is imperative that the terms and conditions meet the necessary rules and regulations as well as the requirements of the donor, the recipient organization and state and federal agencies. Appropriate celebratory and recognition events are indicated with certain gifts, for example, endowed chairs; named and endowed clinical programs; scholarships and the naming of buildings (including hospitals and schools of medicine). All processes need to be conducted with efficiency, be mistake free and cost effective. In our recently completed capital campaign, the medical sciences spent approximately two cents for every dollar collected for expenses, which was reflective of appropriate frugality, a lean organization and the many large gifts comprising the $1,750,000,000 total collected over the ten year period.

Finally apropos of Principle Six, the component parts that comprise the AHC which include departments, divisions, centers and programs, need to be effectively, professionally and enthusiastically served by the Development Office to prevent any feeling of "second degree citizenship" in the organization.

Through all of this, the leader is once again key. Should he or she lack interest, be inappropriately shy about asking for donations (which is an acquired skill) and fail to establish one's self in the community, it will lessen the effectiveness of the Development Office and the entire development effort of the institution.

To summarize what I learned on the job regarding fund-raising I have constituted Levey's Eight Principles for Fund-Raising shown below.

Principle One: You need respected people in the community introducing you to the people of influence and affluence in the community.

Principle Two: Be thoroughly prepared when soliciting a donor.

Principle Three: Ask for what you need; don't try to guess what the donor will give.

Principle Four: Be patient, keep trying and never give up.

Principle Five: Donors to AHCs expect quid pro quo for their gifts: access to the best medical care.

Principle Six: Don't compete with the faculty.

Principle Seven: Philanthropy is a contact sport.

Principle Eight: Create a first-rate Office of Development.

CHAPTER FIFTEEN

EVERY LEADER NEEDS A JOKE

One of the attributes of success in leadership is having a sense of humor. In Chapter Three I noted this attribute on the personal value scale but deferred discussion until this later chapter. A sense of humor is a very tangible and even critical attribute serving many purposes for a successful leader. Perhaps most important is that it humanizes the leader when their sense of humor is revealed in the appropriate time, place and context; making people laugh, even in a time of crisis and tension, can relax the atmosphere in a room and enable the participants to hopefully reach better solutions. The leader of any major organization is called upon for multiple speaking engagements during the ordinary workweek and an abundant schedule of evening engagements with community and national organizations.

It is good for the people in the audience, who either relate directly to the leader or have an interest in helping the AHC, to embrace the vision of the leader. The leader should project being thoughtful, serious and one who can set a proper tone by using a funny story or two.

Over the thirty years of my career in a leadership position in academic health centers, I have accumulated approximately 300 jokes and an equal number of one-liners. Unfortunately, or fortunately, I had multiple sources for the jokes including, most recently, jokes that were sent to me by others via e-mail. With apologies to the originators of these jokes, I hope they realize that they have brought great joy and much laughter to people who have heard me speak.

In the present chapter, I have included a sampling of these jokes many of them in the broad category of healthcare. Also, as a physician, I have included some good natured stories of lawyers — a time honored indulgence of physicians; lawyers have a similar panoply of jokes about the medical profession. Where possible, the one-liners I have used can either be attributed to Henry "Henny" Youngman or Rodney Dangerfield both of whom were considered the kings of the one-liners during their decades of entertaining.

I hope this sampling of jokes will serve the reader, present and future, and add a new dimension to the many leaders we have both in medicine, business and other walks of life. An important piece of advice for the present and future leaders is that one has to know his or her audience before venturing into a risqué joke. Additionally, you should always do a trial run of your jokes on your friends in the office or your spouse; this will serve the dual purpose of perfecting your delivery and obtaining opinions regarding whether a joke should or should not be told. Similarly, ethnic humor requires a sensitive touch and should not be used if it will offend. Finally, the way you tell the joke, its delivery and your enjoying the joke is key for the response to the joke; relax and be natural.

I hope you enjoy the jokes!!!

ACADEMIC LEADERSHIP/ADMINISTRATION

Major US Research University
Discovers New Element

The heaviest element known to science was recently discovered by investigators at a major US research university. The element, tentatively named Administratium, has no protons or electrons and thus has an atomic number of zero. However, it does have one neutron, 125 assistant neutrons, 75 vice neutrons and 111 assistant vice neutrons. This gives it an atomic mass of 312.

These 312 particles are held together by a force that involves the continuous exchange of meson-like particles called morons. It is also surrounded by vast quantities of lepton-like particles called peons.

Since it has no electrons, Administratium is inert. However, it can be detected chemically as it impedes every reaction it comes in contact with. According to the discoverers, a minute amount of Administratium caused one reaction to take over four days to complete when it would have normally occurred in less than one second.

Administratium has a normal half-life of approximately three years, at which time it does not decay, but instead undergoes a reorganization in which assistant neutrons, vice neutrons and assistant vice neutrons exchange places.

In fact, an Administratium sample's mass actually INCREASES over time, since with each reorganization some of the morons inevitably become neutrons, forming new isotopes.

This characteristic of moron promotion leads some scientists to speculate that perhaps Administratium is spontaneously formed whenever morons reach a certain quantity in concentration. This hypothetical quantity is referred to as "critical morass."

Prepare Three Envelopes

The business of being a chairman is high risk with an average professional life span of about four years. There is a famous story of a chairman who takes a job at a prestigious university in the northeast and the first day on the job his administrative assistant tells him that the previous chairman left three envelopes in the lower right hand drawer of his desk to be opened only in the event of extreme difficulties. Well — things go well for the chairman for the first six months during the usual honeymoon period, and then he begins to have a great deal of difficulty. A few of his division chiefs begin to give him a hard time about some of his policies, the students are unhappy with the teaching program, and a few residents are not performing very well. Finally, he is sitting at his desk one day and decides he better reach into the right hand drawer and pull out the first envelope. He opens it and reads the inscription that says "Blame your predecessor." So he blames the previous chairman and sure enough that works and within two months all of his problems are resolved and for about eighteen months things actually go pretty well. Then he begins to have trouble with his dean who is giving him some problems with the budget. He has more trouble with the students and house staff and one day, while very frustrated, he remembers the envelopes, opens the lower right hand drawer, and pulls out envelope number two. Envelope number two says, "Reorganize the department." So, he reorganizes the department, replaces a few of the division chiefs, brings in some new recruits and sure enough — corrects all of the problems and everything goes beautifully. About two years later, the department deteriorates even worse than before. He's having terrible problems with the dean, budget reveals he is in deficit, the students are unhappy with his teaching program and his office administrator walks out. Totally frustrated, he decides it is time to open the lower right hand drawer and open envelope three. So, he opens the drawer and opens up the envelope and reads the note. It says one simple line — "Prepare three envelopes."

HEALTHCARE

Seventy-Five-Year-Old's Annual Checkup

A seventy-five-year-old man goes to the doctor for his annual check-up. The doctor finishes and says, "George, you're in excellent health. As a matter of fact, you're in an amazing state of health. In my clinical experience, it must have to do with heredity. How old was your father when he died?" George said, "Who said my father is dead? He is 95 and in excellent health." "Well," the physician said, "How old was your grandfather when he died?" George said, "Who says he is dead? He is 115 and getting married next week to a twenty-year-old girl." The doctor said, "He is 115 and getting married to a twenty-year-old girl! Why would he want to do that at his age?" George responded, "Who says he wants to?"

The New American Healthcare System

I hurt my hand the other day and decided to go to an Urgent Care Center to have my hand examined. I walked in the front door and there was no one there — there were no physicians, no nurses and no physician assistants. I looked around and saw two doors. Over one door was written "illness" and over the other "injury." Well, I thought for a moment and said, "I injured my hand, I guess I'll open that door and go in." So I entered and still there was no one there. But as I looked around I saw there were two more doors and on the first door was the word "emergency" and the second door had "non-emergency." Well, I knew this wasn't exactly a traditional emergency so I opened the non-emergency door. Once again, there was no one in the room but I saw two more doors and on one door was written the word "trunk" and on the other was written the word "appendage." This was an easy decision because I knew it was my hand that I hurt, so I opened the "appendage" door and walked in. Once more there was no one in the room, but there were two more doors. On one door was written "bleeding" and the other door "not bleeding." Well this again was an easy decision because about an hour or so ago my hand was bleeding but now it wasn't — so I opened the "non-bleeding door." And when I opened that door, in front of me was the parking lot. So I walked over to my car and there on the windshield was a bill!!

Medical Advice

I was working around the house and I sprained my wrist and wasn't really feeling very well so I went to my doctor. The doctor looked at it, moved it around and said, "Well, it hurts when you move it, obviously there's a little swelling, I think you sprained your wrist. What I recommend is that you put hot compresses on it and it should be better in no time." I said thank you, went home and started putting hot compresses on it. A couple of days went by and it still wasn't feeling right. I was walking outside, flexing my wrist, I had the hot compress on and my gardener saw what I was doing and he said, "What's the matter, doc?" I said, "Well, I sprained my wrist and I've been putting these hot compresses on and it just isn't feeling any better." He said, "Of course not, you sprained your wrist, you should be putting ice on it." I said, "Gee, my doctor told me to put heat on it." He said, "Oh no, no, no, put ice on it." So I went back into the house, I put ice on it, I used it a lot that day and within 24 hours my wrist was better. Well, I was a little bit annoyed that my doctor hadn't prescribed correctly for me, so I went to see him the next day. He said, "How's the wrist feeling?" I said, "Feels perfect, but not because of you." I said, "I put hot compresses on it and my wrist didn't get any better, and my gardener took a look at it and he said to put ice on it and within 24 hours it was better." The doctor looked at me and said, "Huh, my gardener recommends heat for sprains."

HMO – Medical Insurance Explained

Q. What does HMO stand for?

A. This is actually a variation of the phrase, "HEY MOE." Its roots go back to a concept pioneered by Moe of the Three Stooges, who discovered that a patient could be made to forget the pain in his foot if he was poked hard enough in the eye.

Q. I just joined an HMO. How difficult will it be to choose the doctor I want?

A. Just slightly more difficult than choosing your parents. Your insurer will provide you with a book listing all the doctors in the plan. The doctors basically fall into two categories — those who are no longer accepting new patients and those who will see you, but are no longer participating in the plan. But don't worry, the remaining doctor who is still in the plan and accepting new patients has an office just a half-day's drive away and a diploma from a third world country.

Q. Do all diagnostic procedures require pre-certification?

A. No. Only those you need.

Q. Can I get coverage for my preexisting conditions?

A. Certainly, as long as they don't require treatment.

Q. What happens if I want to try alternative forms of medicine?

A. You'll need to find alternative forms of payment.

Q. My pharmacy plan only covers generic drugs, but I need the name brand. I tried the generic medication, but it gave me a stomach ache. What should I do?

A. Poke yourself in the eye.

Q. What if I'm away from home and I get sick?

A. You really shouldn't do that.

Q. I think I need to see a specialist, but my doctor insists he can handle my problem. Can a general practitioner really perform a heart transplant right in his/her office?

A. Hard to say, but considering that all you're risking is the $20 co-payment, there's no harm in giving it a shot.

Q. Will health care be different in the next century?

A. No, but if you call right now, you might get an appointment by then.

Angel and the Dean's Reward

An angel appears at a faculty meeting and tells the dean that in return for his unselfish and exemplary behavior, the Lord will reward him with his choice of infinite wealth, wisdom or beauty. Without hesitating, the dean selects infinite wisdom. "Done!" says the angel and disappears in a cloud of smoke and a bolt of lightning. Now all heads turn toward the dean who sits surrounded in a halo of light. Finally, one of his colleagues whispers, "Say something." The dean looks at them and says, "I should have taken the money."

An Analyst and His Therapist

An analyst had a very nervous patient that he had been seeing for over eight years. Finally, after concluding that further therapy was not needed, he said to the patient, "Okay, this is the last session; the therapy is over, and you are not to come back here anymore." The patient nervously said, "You know how fragile I am. What will I do if I have another attack?" "If you have another attack, work it out, and call me in the morning," replied the therapist. Sure enough, the very next day the patient called the analyst, "I had a terrible attack last night — really awful." The therapist asked, "What happened?" The patient replied, "I had a terrible dream, really frightening. I dreamt you were my mother!" The analyst asked, "Then what happened?" The patient answered, "After I calmed down, I got out of bed and went downstairs for breakfast — I had a cup of coffee and a doughnut." The analyst said, "You call that a breakfast?"

Talking Frog

A woman is walking along the beach and as she is walking, she sees a frog. The frog says to her, "Kiss me and I'll become an orthopaedic surgeon, marry you, and you'll be rich and live the lush life." She bends down, picks the frog up, puts the frog in her pocket and continues to walk along the beach. In the meantime, this gentleman is watching her and doesn't quite understand what is happening. He walks over to her and says, "I heard what the frog said to you but you put the frog in your pocket and you kept walking along. Why? The frog said if you kissed him he would become an orthopaedic surgeon and you would be wealthy and live in fine style." The woman looked at him and said, "In this era of healthcare reform, I think I am better off with a talking frog, than an orthopaedic surgeon."

SCIENCE

Cloning

A physician who heads a clinic is very, very busy seeing patients and doing administration. He is finding that he cannot keep up with this work or function efficiently as a doctor. Therefore, he decides to clone himself in order to ease his workload. After the cloning procedure is completed and his clone is working in the clinic, he finds life much easier. He has more time for patients and is doing his administration more efficiently since it's shared. But after a month, problems begin to develop. The clone is very aggressive, highly outspoken and uses foul language. A few weeks go by and he continues to insult people and offend their sensibilities with his vulgar language. One day the physician calls the clone into his office and tells him that his behavior is unsatisfactory and the clone responds with a flurry of vulgar words and the physician takes him and throws him out the window, down fifteen floors. Ten minutes later the police come and say he's under arrest. The physician says, "You can't arrest me, I just killed myself." The police say, "Oh yes we can." He says, "On what grounds?" The police replied, "For making an obscene clone fall."

LAWYERS

Engineer Joke

An engineer dies and reports to the pearly gates. Saint Peter checks his dossier and says, "Ah, you're an engineer — you're in the wrong place."

So the engineer reports to the gates of hell and is let in.

Pretty soon, the engineer becomes dissatisfied with the level of comfort in hell, and starts designing and building improvements. After a while they've got air conditioning and flush toilets and escalators, and the engineer is a pretty popular guy.

One day God calls Satan up on the telephone and says with a sneer, "So, how's it going down there in hell?" Satan replies, "Hey, things are going great. We've got air conditioning and flush toilets and escalators, and there's no telling what this engineer is going to come up with next."

God replies, "What?!?! You've got an engineer? That's a mistake — he should never have gotten down there, send him up here!" Satan says, "No way. I like having an engineer on the staff, and I'm keeping him." God says, "Send him back up here or I'll sue!" Satan laughs uproariously and answers, "Yeah right! And just where are YOU going to get a lawyer?"

Lawyer, Accountant and Physician

Three men — a lawyer, a Jewish accountant and a Hindu physician — are driving on a country road. The car breaks down and they see a farm house and go over and knock on the door. They ask the farmer if it would be alright if they spend the night since it's late and cold and the car has broken down. The farmer says, "Well, I don't have any room in the farm house, but two of you could sleep in the shed and the barn will accommodate one. So the three of them discuss it and the Jewish accountant says, "I'll sleep in the barn. I don't mind." And the other two go into the shed. After the two men in the shed get settled, they hear a knock on the door and it's the Jewish accountant. He tells them, "I'm sorry, I can't sleep in the barn. There's a pig in there and since I'm kosher, it's impossible to stay there with the pig."

So the Hindu physician says, "Well, that's ok. I'm happy to sleep in the barn." He leaves and goes into the barn. In only a few minutes, there's a knock on the door of the shed and it's the Hindu physician. He says, "I'm sorry, I can't stay in the barn. As you know, cows are sacred to Hindus and there's a cow in the barn." Finally the lawyer agrees to sleep in the barn and several minutes later there's a knock on the door of the shed and its the farmer, with the cow and the pig.

Wealthy Man's Last Request

A very wealthy man is dying and as he is dying, he gathers his three best friends around his bedside. They are his priest, his physician and his lawyer. He tells them he wants them to promise him that they will fulfill his last wish. They all ask what the wish is and he says, "I'm not going to tell you. I want you to first promise me that you will fulfill my wish." They say to their good friend, "Well, certainly, that's the least we can do for you." He says "Good. My wish is as follows: When I die you will each be handed an envelope containing $100,000. I want each of you to throw it into my grave after they lower me into the ground." They think this is a strange request but, nevertheless, they say, "We definitely promise we will do this." So the wealthy man dies. At the time of the funeral, each of them throws the envelope into the grave. As they are walking out of the cemetery, the priest stops and says, "Listen, this is on my conscience. I have to admit this to you. I, in a way, violated the promise. I thought it was ridiculous to throw an envelope containing $100,000 into the grave, so I took $25,000 out to help support our special fund for the poor and the needy. Certainly $25,000 out of the $100,000 to help these unfortunate people can be understood and forgiven." Then the doctor says, "Well, now that you have confessed, let me also admit that I violated the promise. Our hospital wing is not completed and we needed some money and I took $50,000 out to complete our new hospital wing." And then the lawyer speaks and says, "Well, I also broke the promise. I opened the envelope and put in a personal check for $100,000."

HEAVEN

Meeting with Saint Peter

Three men died and went to heaven and as they were being processed, they met with Saint Peter. Saint Peter said to the first man, before we decide your mode of transportation in heaven, I have to ask you a question: "How faithful were you to your wife?" The first man answered, "I was very faithful, I never had an affair." Saint Peter said, "That's very good, you get to drive around heaven in a white Cadillac Seville." Saint Peter then turned to the second man, "How faithful were you to your wife?" The second man answered, "Well — I wasn't totally faithful. I cheated on her once or twice." Saint Peter said, "Then you get to drive the Ford." Finally, he asked the third man, "How faithful were you to your wife?" And the third man answered, "Well, I really wasn't very faithful and about once a month I cheated on my wife." Saint Peter said, "Then you get to drive the motorcycle." After a few days, the man in the Ford and the man on the motorcycle met and were talking together when, all of a sudden, the first man in the white Cadillac Seville drove up and he looked absolutely terrible. He had the most unhappy face they had ever seen. They went over to the car and said, "What's the matter? You look so unhappy. How can you be unhappy in heaven driving a white Cadillac Seville?" The man looked at them and said, "I was driving around heaven the other day and I looked out the window and there was my wife on a pair of roller skates!"

GENERAL

Monk at a Monastery

A monk enters the monastery. At the time of entry, he was informed of the rule that you were only allowed to say two words every five years. The first five years go by and he approaches the director of the monastery and says, "Food cold." The director says, "O.K. We'll look into that." Another five years goes by and the monk again approaches the director and says, "Bed hard."

The director says, "Well, we'll look into that and try to take care of it." Another five years go by and the monk goes to the director of the monastery and says, "I quit," to which the director of the monastery says, "Good riddance. All you've done since you got here is complain."

Soup or Sex

An elderly gentleman was about to celebrate his 75th birthday. His wife had passed away several years earlier and he had spent the time since then alone. His son decided that he was going to make his father's 75th birthday occasion something he would never forget. On the morning of his birthday, the man heard a knock on his door. He opened the door to find the most gorgeous woman, dressed in a very revealing dress. She said to him, "Your son sent me. I'm here to give you super sex!" The old man looked at her for a moment and then replied, "I'll take the soup."

"NAN" Organization

A gentleman gets on a plane and is flying first class. He sits down in a seat next to a very attractive woman and notices that she has a locket around her neck which has the letters NAN on it. Just then the stewardess makes an announcement that the plane is going to be delayed because of some repairs that have to be made but that they will begin to take drink orders. She comes over to where the gentleman is sitting and asks him what he would like to drink and he says, "I'll have a Beefeater martini, thank you," and looks over and says, "Nan, what would you like?" She orders a scotch and water and says to him, "But my name isn't Nan, it is Donna." The man says, "Oh, I'm so embarrassed! I didn't realize. I just assumed your name was Nan because of the letters on your locket." And she says, "Oh no, that is not my name — that's stands for the organization I belong to." And he says, "Oh, what organization is that?" And she says, "The National Association of Nymphomaniacs." And he says, "The National Association of Nymphomaniacs? I've never heard of that one!" And she says, "Yes. It is a very active group." And he says, "Oh, I'm sure it must be a very interesting organization. Tell me — since you are a member you must know a great deal about sex and men. Who are your favorite lovers?" She thinks for a moment and then says, "Cowboys, number one; they are so rugged and virile, and the Jewish men, number two, because they are so considerate and sensitive." Then she says, "By the way, what's your name?" And he says, "Hopalong Goldberg!"

Sophie and Sadie

Two elderly Jewish women, Sophie and Sadie, make a pact that the first one who dies will call the other one on the phone and let them know what life is like after death. Well — Sophie dies and Sadie begins her vigil by the phone to await Sophie's phone call. Days, then several weeks go by, and no phone call. Finally one day, the phone rings, Sadie picks it up and it's Sophie. She says, "Sophie, I have been waiting for your call. Tell me! What's it like after death?" Sophie says, "Well, it's not bad. I get up in the morning, I eat a salad, have a little sex, and then rest until lunch. I then get up, have lunch, eat a little salad, have some sex, and then I rest until dinner. At dinner I have a nice salad, I have some more sex, and then I go to bed until breakfast the next day." And Sadie says, "This is absolutely wonderful!! Heaven sounds terrific!" And Sophie says, "Heaven? Who's in heaven? I'm a rabbit in New Jersey."

Memorial Stone

A woman's husband dies. He had left $30,000 to be used for an elaborate funeral. After everything is done at the funeral home and cemetery, she tells her closest friend that "there is absolutely nothing left of the $30,000."

The friend asks, "How can that be?"

The widow says, "Well, the funeral cost was $6,500. And, of course, I made a donation to the church — that was $500, and I spent another $500 for the wake, food and drinks — you know. The rest went for the memorial stone."

The friend says, "$22,500 for the memorial stone? My God, how big is it?"

The widow says, "Four and a half carats."

Betty Crocker

A husband is at home watching a football game when his wife interrupts, "Honey, could you fix the light in the hallway? It's been flickering for weeks now." He looks at her and says angrily, "Fix the light? Now? Does it look like I have a G.E. logo printed on my forehead? I don't think so." The wife replies, "Well then, could you fix the fridge door? It won't close right." To which he replied, "Fix the fridge door? Does it look like I have Westinghouse written on my forehead? I don't think so." "Fine," she says, "Then could you at least fix the steps to the front door? They're about to break." "I'm not a darn carpenter and I don't want to fix the steps," he says, "Does it look like I have Ace Hardware written on my forehead? I don't think so. I've had enough of you. I'm going to the bar!" So he goes to the bar and drinks for a couple of hours. He starts to feel guilty about how he treated his wife, and decides to go home and help out. As he walks up to the house, he notices the steps are already fixed. As he enters the house, he sees the hall light is working. As he goes to get a beer, he notices the fridge door is fixed. "Honey, how'd all this get fixed?" She said, "Well, when you left I sat outside and cried. Just then a nice young man asked me what was wrong and I told him. He offered to do all the repairs and all I had to do was either go to bed with him or bake a cake." He said, "So, what kind of cake did you bake him?" She replied, "Hellooooo… do you see Betty Crocker written on my forehead?"

ONE LINER JOKES:

Thank you, Henry "Henny" Youngman!!

A doctor gave a man six months to live. The man couldn't pay his bill, so he gave him another six months.

The doctor called Mrs. Cohen saying, "Mrs. Cohen, your check came back." Mrs. Cohen answered, "So did my arthritis!"

A man goes to his doctor for an annual checkup. He comes back a week later to learn the results and asks, "How am I doing doctor?" The doctor says, "You'll live to be sixty!" "I AM SIXTY!" "See, what'd I tell you?"

A doctor says to a man, "You want to improve your love life? You need to get some exercise. Run ten miles a day." Two weeks later, the man called the doctor. The doctor asks, "How is your love life since you've been running?" "I don't know, I'm 140 miles away!"

A man goes to a psychiatrist, "Nobody listens to me!" The doctor says, "Next!"

Nurse: "Doctor, the man you just gave a clean bill of health to dropped dead right as he was leaving the office." Doctor: "Turn him around; make it look like he was walking in."

I told my dentist my teeth are turning yellow. He told me to wear a brown necktie.

A priest is sent to Alaska. A bishop goes up to visit one year later. The bishop asks, "How do you like it up here?" The priest says, "If it wasn't for my Rosary, and two martinis a day, I'd be lost. Bishop, would you like a martini?" "Yes." "Rosary, get the bishop a martini!"

Last week I saw my psychiatrist. I told him, "Doc, I keep thinking I'm a dog." He told me to get off his couch.

CHAPTER SIXTEEN

I'D DO IT AGAIN

I am frequently asked the question as to whether or not I would do this job again and I invariably tell the people that the answer is: I most certainly would. Although the simple answer "yes", expresses the way I feel, the response is more complicated, especially if the person asking the question aspires to a leadership position. Allow me to expand on the answer and make some observations that are pertinent to the answer "yes;" these observations focus on experience, preparation and motivation.

I believed I was fully prepared to become vice chancellor for Medical Sciences and dean of the David Geffen School of Medicine at UCLA having learned from two of the master mentors in my career; Dr. Thomas

Detre who oversaw the entire Academic Health Center at the University of Pittsburgh, a position similar to mine at UCLA, and Dr. Roy Vagelos, the CEO and chairman of Merck. Both of them had an amazing vision for their respective organizations; they both assumed command of organizations that had enormous potential and needed change and firm leadership. Both leaders were tenacious, indefatigable, civil, courteous to all and, at the same time, strong-willed and driven to achieve their objectives. Neither became bogged down in minutiae, but knew how to keep their eyes focused on the big picture. I learned good lessons by just observing these leaders of their respective organizations.

In Chapters One and Three, I recounted the admonition from Dr. Detre — when we were discussing my future career — that I needed one more step in experience to head an Academic Health Center beyond being a chairman of medicine. He was correct, of course, and I took his advice with considerable trepidation, but when Merck came calling and offered me the position of senior vice president for Medical and Scientific Affairs, I accepted the job much to the amazement of my colleagues in academia. Merck became, for me, a three year sabbatical and I learned from Dr. Vagelos how to run a large, complicated, result-oriented organization; to endure the pressures of the job; to never lose your cool and to never fail to admit your mistakes or lose sight of the goals and core mission of the greater organization. I improved my communication skills in part by observing Dr. Vagelos, and in part by Merck's mandatory face-to-face meetings with the employees who reported to you. I also learned the importance from both mentors of surrounding yourself with extraordinarily talented people who also shared the same principles for which you stood.

In addition to the University of Pittsburgh and Merck, my early career, discussed in Chapter One, provided exceptional training at first-rate places; the University of Medicine and Dentistry of New Jersey, the Department of Biological Chemistry at Harvard Medical School, the Massachusetts General Hospital, the National Institutes of Health and the University of Miami School of Medicine, where I was a Howard Hughes Medical Investigator. My diverse experiences with my various positions in academia were ideal for the job I was about to begin at UCLA. In essence my career, like many CEOs, started at the bottom and worked my way up the ladder from job to job each one being a step higher than the next so that at the end, I thoroughly understood the mission and complexities of an Academic Medical Center or Academic Health Center and had dealt with many of the issues. I was also fortunate to arrive in Los Angeles shortly after the earthquake which provided me not only with a great opportunity but a faculty, administration, chancellor and executive vice chancellor all of whom were looking for leadership in the medical sciences at a difficult and challenging time for UCLA. Therefore, the diversity of my background was ideal and one of the major reasons for the success I enjoyed at UCLA.

Lastly, I was motivated; I unequivocally wanted to assume the responsibilities for a large, vibrant Academic Health Center. I knew beyond any doubt this would be the capstone of my career and I was not afraid I would fail in the process because of my sense of preparedness. My qualified "yes," therefore, recognizes the fact that if you are prepared, experienced and motivated, the chances for success are good, but if you aren't, the chances of success diminish. When Dr. Detre said I needed one more preparatory experience (Merck), he was correct so that when I was actually offered the position at UCLA, I was, by preparation, experience and motivation, ready for what lay ahead.

I would also do this job again because there is so much opportunity to do good as a CEO of a major academic health center. The reward for doing well is to make a difference in your life in a critical area for our society, i.e., healthcare. In addition to the university embracing new leadership, new ideas and new challenges, the community also embraced a new leader. The support I was able to generate from the community was really special, and as a side benefit, provided an essential alternate source of financial support that remained strong and constant. Every leader in an AHC needs this kind of support. The people in the Los Angeles community are amazing and many played a role in my personal success and more importantly, to fulfilling the greater mission of UCLA's hospital system and School of Medicine.

Anyone who entertains thoughts of leadership must also be aware of the incredible work effort that is required to be a CEO of a major organization. The time demands are phenomenal; the number of evenings one must be on the dinner circuit was even beyond my expectation. However, being on that circuit and frequently having to speak to the audiences built relationships and carried the UCLA message as it would for any organization where its CEO is represented at these functions. In general, the time that the leader has to spend is also something that you must experience to appreciate. One time in New Jersey one of my friends told me about the chairman and CEO of Hess Oil, who was an incredibly hard worker and expected no less from the employees and the company. The employees used to say that the name of the company, Hess, stood for holidays, evenings, Saturdays and Sundays. Based on my experiences in my position, this certainly was true for me and I am sure this extends to anyone else leading a major organization. Without any doubt, you have to be willing to expend the effort in order to successfully fulfill the mission of the organization, address the problems, achieve the goals and do the daily things that have to be done. Considering the simplified mission of an Academic Health Center including research, patient care, training and community, success means you have done something that is noble and has meaningfully contributed to our society. Implementing a curriculum for the students to provide a better learning experience is very rewarding if it is done well; leading to better training and better physicians and providing the public with quality healthcare. Recruiting the best and brightest physicians and scientists improves the overall environment of the institution and ultimately translates to better clinical care by bringing the frontier of medical science to the patients. New programs, new buildings, superb faculty and students ensures that the AHC not only acquires a better reputation, but becomes recognized as an important pillar of the local community, state and nation, making healthcare better because of your achievements.

As I reflect back on my fifteen years as vice chancellor and dean, I have been blessed to have been given the position, and especially at a time of need for UCLA. Given all that was accomplished, I am satisfied that I did my best and that I, and everyone on my team, changed the course of history for UCLA's Academic Health Center. I have had a storybook life and UCLA was a true capstone of my career. In what other career and what other medical complex could I have so positively affected people's lives and our society in the greater Los Angeles area? So the answer to the question of "would I do it again" remains an emphatic yes. I hope this book provides a helpful source of information to present and future leaders, which would be the icing on the cake. A cadre of strong, experienced and qualified leaders in our AHCs will be a prerequisite as we navigate a dramatically changing healthcare system in the years ahead.

FACULTY MEETING PRESENTATION

SEPTEMBER 29, 1994

INTRODUCTION

Good afternoon, ladies and gentlemen. It is an honor for me to stand before you as the newly appointed provost for the Medical Sciences and dean of the School of Medicine. This is truly one of the world's outstanding institutions and we can be justifiably proud of our medical school, research units and hospitals, all of which are held in great respect. I would like to use the time today to outline the various challenges and opportunities we face during this period of extraordinary change in which our healthcare system is being reformed, research funding growing ever tighter, financial support from the state declining, reimbursement for both hospitals and physicians decreasing, tuition rising and renovation of old facilities and new construction of laboratories becoming a capital emergency. Consolidation of the duties of the provost and dean should and must enable us to reexamine and optimize the finances of the entire UCLA Medical Science enterprise permitting optimization of resources to support the academic mission. We must develop appropriate clinical programs and strategies; foster programmatic initiatives across the various schools of the undergraduate campus as well as the Schools of the Health Sciences including Dentistry, Public Health and Nursing; develop new and innovative educational programs for students and post graduate trainees; enhance the activities of the Development Office, enabling it to have a more focused and visible role in fund-raising; provide critically needed new and/or renovated laboratory space; harmonize the activities of the hospital and medical school and last but not least, enhance working relationships with the Faculty Executive Committee and the University Senate as we assume a more unitary perspective of our university community and its strengths, resources and needs.

PROVOST/DEANS OFFICE

In my role as provost, I report to the executive vice chancellor. I have direct responsibility for the Medical Center Hospital and the Neuropsychiatric Hospital, therefore, Dr. Raymond Schultz and Dr. Don Rockwell report directly to me. I also have responsibility for the eight Organized Research Units which include the Mental Retardation Research Unit, the AIDS Institute, the Molecular Science Institute, Crump Institute, Jules Stein Eye Institute, the Brain Research Institute, the Jonsson Cancer Center and Neuropsychiatric Institute. The dean of the School of Medicine reports to the provost, although for the foreseeable future, the positions will be unified. The Schools of Nursing and Public Health will not report to the provost, until such time as the provost relinquishes the position of the dean of the School of Medicine. I am comfortable with this arrangement. However, it will not deter us from cross-institutional, programmatic planning and attempts to reduce duplicative services in order to operate more cost effectively.

The provost's office and activities are and will be funded by new negotiated revenue, the hospitals and, ultimately, by utilizing some of the cost savings produced by central fiscal oversight. The office activities will not take needed funds from academic programs. Central to the workings of the provost's office is the appointment of a vice provost for Finance/ Administration with broad oversight and authority for budgetary reform; a vice provost for Medical Affairs, who will have major responsibility for long-range planning and development and a vice provost for Development who will oversee our fund-raising activities. Two other areas reporting to the provost are also depicted on the organizational chart. One is a special advisor to the provost for Clinical Affairs who will serve as a close liaison to the UCLA Medical Group as well as to the hospital as we enter this era of healthcare reform and attempt to develop primary care networks and new relationships with other area hospitals. The Board of Advisors for Medical Sciences Development Programs will consist of a blue ribbon panel of individuals committed to providing, directly and indirectly, the philanthropic resources that will be necessary to accomplish the broad goals of the Medical School Organized Research Units, the Medical Center and Neuropsychiatric Hospitals.

One of the challenges of this new structure will be to ensure that you, the faculty, will not be confronted with another impossible layer of bureaucracy that will consume needed dollars for academic programs. I have met with Glenn Langer and others and am fully aware of the perception that the dean's office has evolved into a highly complex structure and is in need of some reform both financial and organizational. I will use the remainder of this academic year to fully understand the workings of the dean's office and personnel. The dean's office is complicated in part because the environment in which we live is complicated and the responsibilities placed upon the dean's office both by need and fiat are extensive. These responsibilities include admissions, Medical Scientist Training Program, Drew and Riverside students, curriculum, student affairs, financial aid, affirmative action programs, continuing medical education programs, postgraduate medical education training programs, affiliate relations, medical school budget, campus wide administrative activities, support of search committees, space development and other matters related to the research enterprise, expeditious appointments and promotion of faculty, grievances, computer programming, library sciences, grants management and personnel. Having recited this long list I am not certain I have covered every responsibility of the dean's office. Nevertheless, I do promise to streamline the organization and to make it run more efficiently.

Several significant changes have been already made to the structure of the dean's office. The administrative position has been combined with that of the senior associate dean for Finance. A number of administrative duties will also be assumed by the vice provost for Finance/Administration and my executive assistant. The position of associate dean for Clinical Affairs has been eliminated. The distribution and assignment of the title assistant dean is under review and a line-by-line review of various internal and external financial commitments assumed by the dean's office is currently taking place. Finally, announcements will be made in the ensuing months regarding individuals appointed to various duties in the provost/dean's office and redefinition of existing job descriptions.

BUDGET

The financial integrity of the entire medical science enterprise will require my diligent oversight. As I noted earlier, the vice provost for Finance/Administration will have as his/her primary responsibility the in-depth review of the entire budget and a mandate to identify areas of waste, duplication and inefficiency. At a time when the state of California is providing a decreased level of support, when reimbursement of both hospitals and physicians is decreasing, when NIH grant funding is increasingly harder to obtain (especially for young investigators), it is not only critical but mandatory that we operate cost effectively and efficiently. For my part, I will scrutinize the dean's office budget and ensure that the operating expenses do not exceed what is required for us to perform the responsibilities outlined earlier. We must set an example with utilization of personnel and fiscal responsibility if I am to be credible when I ask you to operate your units in that same manner — and I will ask. Department Chairs, Division Directors and other administrative heads must utilize their resources to the fullest. All resources must be available as part of the greater available budget, to support the operation as a whole. "One for all and all for one" is as true today as it ever was and it must be one of our guiding principles. Among our diverse group, some units are stronger than others and have available opportunities that some do not have for funding. The rich and strong must help units poorer and deserving of supplemental funding.

The dean's office cannot do everything — it simply is not possible. On the positive side, we are still richly endowed compared to many private institutions in the United States. Support from the state of California is still relatively strong; the UCLA hospitals under the able stewardships of Drs. Raymond Schultz and Don Rockwell are on sound financial ground and contribute substantially to the academic mission of UCLA. For the most part, the practice plans are doing well. Grant funding remains strong and the Howard Hughes Medical Institute is a godsend. We must build on these, plan for the future by new programmatic initiatives and operate in a responsible and cost effective manner.

DEVELOPMENT

This discussion provides a nice segue for the next topic — development. If we are to make UCLA's School of Medicine and the Medical Sciences the best they can be, we must expand our development activities to unprecedented levels of success. Funding for substantive renovations of old facilities, construction of new facilities for laboratory research, teaching and innovative clinical programs, endowment for Chairs, discretionary funds to seed new programmatic efforts and investigators in transition will require the support of the private sector including individual donors and industry. We are fortunate to be situated in an area where there is so much goodwill toward UCLA. Many individuals and corporations have supported the greater academic mission of UCLA in the past and with our appropriate attention will continue to do so in the future. We must, however, take fund-raising to unparalleled levels of success. We are fortunate to have exceptional individuals such as Associate Dean for Development and Community Relations, Mitchell Covell, and Vice Provost for Development, Mike Eicher and their staff. I have already begun work in this area. During the transition period, I had substantive discussions with potential benefactors. I will be examining the structure and mission of the board of visitors and board of advisors and attempt to harmonize these functions with the broadened role of the provost. As I noted earlier, I will be developing a special blue ribbon committee to serve as a board of advisors to the provost for long range resource planning and development. The major role of this committee will be to translate our financial needs for a wide variety of capital projects and academic programs into reality by broadly increasing the donor base for the Medical Sciences at UCLA.

In order for the Development Office to be successful it will require the cooperation and active participation of the faculty. You must help us identify key donors relevant to your area of expertise and interest. Where necessary, you will be called upon to articulate the need for the initiative to the donor(s). I must insist on coordinated efforts through the Development Office in order to prevent diffuse and ineffective efforts at fund-raising and to ensure that individual donors, groups or corporations are not confronted with a conflicting menu of requests. The net result of our concentrated efforts will hopefully be an increased number of endowed chairs, a new Molecular Neuroscience Building housing the programs in neuroscience and of sufficient size to accommodate other key research programs such as genetics; new teaching space for innovative programs; funds to remodel existing space and the seeding of other programmatic initiatives such as genetics, including gene therapy and diabetes to name just a few.

STATUS OF SEARCHES FOR CHAIRPERSONS AND CENTER DIRECTORS

1. PEDIATRICS

Thanks to an extraordinary effort by the Search Committee chaired by Dr. Dennis Slamon and the help of Drs. Sid Golub and Dave Meyer, the Pediatrics search was officially concluded in early August. Dr. Edward McCabe, a distinguished pediatrician from Baylor University School of Medicine, will join the faculty on October 15, 1994. Dr. McCabe was co-director of the Molecular Genetics Institute at Baylor and will play a key role in our overall genetics effort at UCLA. I became involved in his recruitment as soon as I accepted my position in early July. Dr. McCabe and I met on two occasions and worked out the various aspects of his recruitment package so neither of us "inherited" the other. I can assure you he is an extraordinarily intelligent, energetic, personable individual who will be a significant leader among the chairpersons and the faculty at large.

UCLA is fortunate to have recruited him. He is a worthy successor to an exceptional chairman, Dr. William Friedman, who made the present department a national power. Dr. McCabe's wife, Linda McCabe, has been hard at work in the Mental Retardation and Research Center since September 1, 1994.

2. PATHOLOGY

The search for the new chairperson of the Department of Pathology has not been brought to a successful conclusion. Two search committees have struggled unsuccessfully over the past 2 – 3 years to recruit a new chairperson. There have been many conflicting issues of science and service that unfortunately could not be resolved. On August 15, 1994, I re-formed the search committee under the direction of Dr. Joe Lane, who agreed to take on this task. In my charge to the committee, I expressly stated that I wanted the department to be headed by someone with a distinguished ongoing record of achievement in scientific research who also understands the clear and important imperative to build a strong and high quality clinical service. Administrative experience, though desirable, is not a prerequisite for the chairperson. This can almost always be provided or learned. I've also met with the Department of Pathology and explained my views. I want the Department of Pathology to be worthy of the UCLA tradition of excellence.

3. ANATOMY/NEUROBIOLOGY

This committee is chaired by Dr. John Mazziotta. It is hard at work, has developed a short list and has initiated arrangements for campus visits by these individuals. Hopefully this search can be concluded and a new chair in place sometime between June 1 and September 1, 1995.

4. GENETICS

A new Department of Genetics will be formed. Clearly all aspects of genetics will be at the frontier in the 21st century and requires us to provide first-rate educational programs for students, residents and physicians beyond the training years; the finest in basic and clinical research and clinical programs such as gene therapy. The dean has committed FTE's, space is being planned to suffice until the Molecular Neuroscience Building is completed and the foundation for developing the complex ground work for an approved graduate program is being developed by Drs. Elizabeth Neufeld and Jake Lusis. I've spoken to many of the concerned parties within the broad umbrella of UCLA and there is a unanimous opinion as to the need for a strong, outside leader in genetics to serve as the department's first chairperson. This search committee is chaired by Jake Lusis and has already begun its work.

5. CANCER CENTER DIRECTOR

The search committee was appointed in August by Dr. Sidney Golub and will be chaired by Dr. Jean deKernion. The committee is hard at work; hopefully its task can be concluded this year.

6. SURGERY SEARCH COMMITTEE

After discussions with Dr. E. Carmack Holmes, interim chair of the Department of Surgery and William Longmire, professor of Surgery, I have delayed appointing a search committee. The department needs a period of reassessment and several key issues central to the department need to be resolved before the recruitment process results in candidates visiting the campus. This is a critical department, central to the success of the Medical Center. It is a department with excellent faculty and strong research and clinical programs, many of which are internationally recognized. I look forward to working with Dr. Holmes, learning more about the department, and hopefully resolving all key issues in a manner fair to all concerned and attracting an equally outstanding leader to succeed Mike Zinner who, unfortunately for us, left to become chair of the Department of Surgery at Harvard.

As you can see, there is a critical need with regard to recruitment and this presents a great opportunity for UCLA and for me. We must not fail. In addition to these recruitments, retirements over the next few years will produce additional openings. Thus there will be a substantial infusion of new people into leadership positions within the Medical School.

COMMUNICATION

One of the important functions of the provost/dean is to communicate and dialogue with the faculty. The job of provost/dean is a complicated one with vast responsibilities. The "buck" clearly stops at my desk and over the next several months and years, I will have many decisions to make, some of them very difficult. Coming from the outside, I will view issues somewhat differently than many of you who have been here for a number of years and some for an entire academic lifetime. I want my decisions to be informed ones — even if you may not agree with all of them. In order to make these decisions, we will have to have an open relationship giving you maximal chance to provide input. Since it is impossible for me to meet one-on-one with everyone who wants to express an opinion on an issue, how will we communicate?

1. I will have at least two general faculty meetings each year—more if necessary. I encourage you to attend. At these sessions, you will have the opportunity to question me. I will also give you the opportunity to prepare written questions for submission prior to the faculty meeting. As with this faculty meeting, the questions may be anonymous. I will then answer them during the question and answer period at the end of the meeting.

2. Starting in October, I will have an ongoing series of lunches with faculty, staff and students which will provide a smaller, more informal forum for getting to know one another. These lunches will be ongoing over the years.

3. We will continue to utilize the format of written communications that has been established in previous administrations.

4. For the first year, I will be scheduling departmental site visits and obtain a broad overview of departmental performance and issues. If this format works, I will attempt to continue these departmental visits on an annual or bi-annual basis.

5. I intend to work closely with the Faculty Executive Committee

and the Faculty Senate and look forward to constructive dialogue on a whole series of issues. For example, some early issues that we will be discussing will include the fate of the Department of Bio-mathematics, a rethinking of departmental structure when indicated, ongoing curriculum reform, new departments, etc.

These are a challenging set of plans for communication given the complexity of my job and the expected noise level. However, I intend to pursue them at the expense of some other activities which are less worthwhile because I believe communication with you, the faculty, is a high priority.

HOSPITALS

Chancellor Young and Executive Vice Chancellor Rich took a bold step by broadening the role of the provost to include responsibility for the Medical Center and the Neuropsychiatric Hospital. Although it increases the complexity of the provost's duties in some ways, it presents an extraordinary opportunity to ensure that the budgets of all units, including the hospitals, can be maximally scrutinized and applied to the greater academic mission. Thus it will be the provost determining to whom and for what resources are provided. This is particularly important with regards to the hospitals in an era characterized by extraordinary pressures on the hospital bottom line. Resources cannot be dispensed from the hospitals without a critical overall view of the academic goals and needs of the Medical School and the financial well-being of the hospitals. I must stress to you the reality that hospitals are no longer "cash-cows." The new realities of the healthcare system with its increasing emphasis on HMOs and systems of capitated care are forcing down reimbursement to hospitals and placing a premium on efficiency. Services are being provided and must be provided by contracts with capitated systems at rates far below those previously charged in an indemnity system. Capitated care now represents greater than 50% of our revenues; indemnity care, less than 10%. The Medical Center recently completed the first phase of Operation Excellence and trimmed $50 million from the expense line. Plans are underway to find another $50 to $75 million in order to bring our costs down to competitive rates in this fiercely competitive marketplace. Unfortunately, we are still among the most expensive hospitals. We must be successful in operating the hospital cost effectively and profitably; there is no other acceptable alternative.

In addition, we must ensure the development of clinical programs that make us different and more attractive in the competitive marketplace. We not only need primary care, we need state of the art programs in various specialties and sub-specialties, including transplantation, cardiovascular diseases, diabetes, geriatrics, oncology, osteoporosis, mental disease, genetics (including gene therapy), to name a few. This will take resources, faculty commitment and an understanding that a faculty with diverse goals and strengths will have to be developed.

The hospitals and the UCLA medical group must continue to be harmonized. Working relationships between the hospitals and the medical group have been vastly improved. The departmental practice groups, as represented by the UCLA medical group, must work in harmony and trust with the hospital. The UCLA medical group must function as a multidisciplinary practice group so we can present ourselves in a competitive fashion by department, program, professional fees and administrative functions to managed care groups. UCLA's clinical departments are in this together and only together will we remain successful.

In this same vein, the hospital and the medical group will be embarking on new adventures such as the development of a primary care network. In a managed care environment with its emphasis on ambulatory services and decreased reliance on hospitals, it will be critical to be part of a health system that will serve two major functions. One is a source of referrals to fill hospital beds. It is generally considered that a population of 100,000 people is required to fill 100 beds of the hospital, a figure altered by certain demographic features such as age of the population. Thus any network of which we are a part will probably require a million people to realistically fill our beds. Second, in addition to ensuring referrals to our hospital, we need primary care sites to serve as training facilities for medical students and postgraduate trainees. Hopefully much of this can be provided in sites directly under the control of full time faculty, but this may not be possible. Certainly all primary care training cannot be accomplished on campus; however, not all sites and personnel are appropriate to teach our medical students and this will be a challenging task to develop the appropriate training in primary care.

Finally, among all of these challenges, several others loom equally large. One, capital must be provided to make the required seismic improvements following the earthquake. We'll hear more about this in the near future once FEMA has decided on the amount of money that will be provided to UCLA because of the earthquake damage and estimates of the seismic soundness of various structures, such as the hospital. It is quite possible that this money will be of such magnitude that a new structure can be constructed which will meet our needs and be seismically sound.

Another challenge will be defining the relationships between the CEOs of the hospital and the provost/dean. I certainly cannot run the hospitals on a daily basis; they certainly will have to accustom themselves to reporting to the chief academic officer of the Medical School and Medical Sciences rather than the executive vice chancellor. It will be of the utmost importance that we work well together. Not working together in a highly effective and beneficial manner is an unacceptable alternative.

BASIC SCIENCE

The basic sciences have provided the critical core for much of our extraordinary research success. The provost/dean must work synergistically with the chairs of the basic sciences departments to ensure their continued success. I am forming a Basic Science Council where the provost and vice provost for Medical Affairs will discuss with the chairs what can be accomplished over the short term to help ensure the research productivity of the departments and equally important, to initiate long range capital programmatic and budgetary planning which will be critically important for the ultimate success of the basic sciences. It is clear that our Development Office must raise necessary funds for renovation of laboratory space and construction of needed new facilities to achieve the long range goals of the basic science departments. There are no other practical and viable alternatives to provide the required funds.

The basic science departments face operational challenges. The new realities of the financial situation in California mandate maximum utilization of our resources. There has been a developing cooperation on many levels between programs in the Medical School and basic science departments in the College of Letters and Sciences. This must continue and will undoubtedly be expanded as we consider programmatic development and departmental structures that best serve the campus at large and its varied teaching and research needs.

The basic science departments must identify ways to operate in a cost effective manner. However I recognize the need for help from the provost/dean since, with one exception, Pharmacology, the departments are unable to generate clinical income which provides extraordinary flexibility for the clinical departments.

Finally, challenges will arise in the area of curriculum. How do we prepare the students for careers in primary care and still provide them adequate knowledge of basic science so critical for the practice of medicine in the 21st century? What do we need to do to stimulate as many students as possible to enter careers in academic medicine since the country clearly needs more physician-scientists? How do we develop more positions for Medical Scientist Training Program students entering the UCLA Medical School class and how do we optimize their success? How do we attract more students into Howard Hughes Medical Institute Fellowships? How do we ensure the success of ACCESS, the graduate program playing such a critical role ensuring the flow of high quality graduate students to the basic sciences? How do we optimize our graduate programs to attract the best and brightest graduate students? I should note that since this presentation was prepared, the dean has contributed an additional $125,000 to ACCESS for 1994 – 95. This program must be kept free of financial difficulties.

Thus, it is clear that many challenges confront the basic science departments, but with appropriate support of the provost/dean these challenges can be overcome.

STUDENTS

The medical students are our greatest natural resource. They also happen to be the reason we are all here. They need to be educated properly, mentored, nurtured and inspired. Our student programs are generally considered to be among the finest in the country, but there are problems.

Fees are inexorably rising. We need to ensure proper student financial aid.

Curriculum needs to be constantly monitored and altered to meet the challenges of a changing healthcare environment. We have a need to train substantially more primary care physicians, but these students must be conversant with the extraordinary advance occurring in the biomedical sciences. The curriculum must continue to be challenging and appropriate for those who select careers in academic medicine and in the various specialties and subspecialties.

UCLA must also concentrate on training more students for careers in academic medicine. With our resources and faculty, we should be a leader in producing physician-scientists including both basic researchers and health services researchers. The STAR Program devised by Linda Demer and Alan Fogelman is an example of what we should be doing in this arena. We must train more residents for careers in science and not to be our competition. We will have to realign our training programs and numbers of trainees to produce more primary care physicians. This will, by necessity, increase the number trainees in general internal medicine, general pediatrics, family medicine and obstetrics/gynecology and fewer in the other specialties.

Students need to be educated as to the workings of the healthcare system and must understand the challenges it will present to them in terms of practice opportunities, financial rewards and various complicated regulatory and administrative issues.

The faculty will need to work hard to ensure that students keep their idealism in this vastly different world that is evolving for the practice of medicine.

The faculty will need to ensure the diversity that has characterized our student body.

We will need to develop appropriate mentors for a diverse student body. This will mandate recruiting an appropriately diverse faculty.

The admissions process will have to be constantly scrutinized to ensure that we continue to attract the very best students to UCLA.

We cannot compromise our excellence.

We will have to optimize our efforts working with our colleagues at Charles R. Drew University of Medicine and Science and the University of California, Riverside to ensure the success of these students including recruitment of outstanding students for these programs and stimulating successful interactions with our faculty.

AFFILIATED HOSITALS

The Medical Sciences have important components off campus, namely, the affiliated hospitals. In my role as provost/dean, I have responsibility for academic programs in these institutions, but no fiduciary responsibilities. Each institution has its own problems; our faculty has concerns some of which are unique to their own environment. Sepulveda was devastated by the earthquake and will no longer have an inpatient service; Harbor General and Olive View are county hospitals that are periodically threatened in the extreme by rumors of closure; Cedars-Sinai is a major clinical competitor of the Medical Center and a large subspecialty-oriented hospital which is beginning to reassess its role in this rapidly changing and competitive health care.

All of our hospitals are key for the overall teaching programs and all have outstanding faculty who contribute to the reputation of UCLA. My involvement will be required on a number of issues such as helping county officials understand the importance of Harbor General and Olive View to the health care of our citizens; central V.A. support of our Veterans Administration hospitals' clinical and research programs and Sepulveda's role post-earthquake; Cedars-Sinai and the Medical Center are/will be exploring all avenues of cooperation, not the least of which are programmatic interactions and training programs.

As provost/dean, I also have academic responsibility for Charles R. Drew University of Medicine and Science. I have met with President Reed Tuckson and have assured him of my complete support for his efforts at Charles R. Drew University of Medicine and Science and its outstanding program. I look forward to serving on its board and working with him and Dean M. Roy Wilson.

Finally, I want to thank all of you for attending today's faculty meeting. I look forward to working with you and will need your help and support. I need to learn about UCLA and its strengths and problems — you need to teach me. I need to make many hard decisions in the years ahead—you need to be prepared for change in an evolutionary, if not, revolutionary period of time for health care, science and fiscal support of academic health centers and universities. As we prepare for next year, no less the next century, we will be stressed and challenged as never before. Together we must develop long-range plans to prepare UCLA to meet these challenges and to be an even greater university in the next century.

Thank you very much.

BIBLIOGRAPHY

Bennis, Warren. *On Becoming a Leader: The Leadership Classic.*
New York: Basic Books, 2009, 254.

Covey, Stephen R. *The 7 Habits of Highly Effective People: Powerful
Lessons in Personal Change.* New York: Fireside Book, 1990, 358.

Exodus 18:14-27. (The Holy Scriptures According to Masoretic Text.)

Kirch, Darrell G. MD, Kevin R. Grigsby, DSW, Wayne W. Zolko, et al.
"Reinventing the Academic Health Center." *Academic Medicine* 80.
No. 11. (November 2005): 980 – 9.

Kouzes, James M., and Barry Z. Posner. *The Leadership Challenge.*
San Francisco: Jossey-Bass, 2002, 202 – 459.

Kurtzman, Joel. *Common Purpose: How Great Leaders Get Organizations to Achieve the Extraordinary.* San Francisco: Jossey-Bass:
2010, 212.

Loop, Floyd D. MD. *Leadership and Medicine.* Gulf Breeze, FL: Fire
Starter Publishing, 2009, 283.

Naylor, C. David. "Leadership in Academic Medicine: Reflections from
Administrative Exile." *Clinical Medicine, Journal of the Royal College
of Physicians* 6, No. 5. (September/October 2006): 488 – 92.

Ramo, Simon, and Ronald Sugar. *Strategic Business Forecasting.* New
York: McGraw-Hill, 2005, 228.

Sample, Steven B. *The Contrarians Guide to Leadership*. San Francisco: Jossey-Bass, 2002, 192.

Schidlow, Daniel V. "Musings on the Nature of Academic Medical Leadership." *Physician Executive* 33, No. 2. (March – April 2007): 32 – 4.

Simone, Joseph V. "Understanding Academic Medical Centers: Simone's Maxims." *Clinical Cancer Research* 5, No. 9. (September 1999): 2281 – 5.

Welch, Jack, and Suzy Welch. *Winning*. New York: HarperCollins, 2005, 373.

Wilson, Emery A., Jay A. Perman and D. Kay Clawson. *Pearls for Leaders in Academic Medicine*. New York: Springer, 2008, 69.

Wooden, John R., and Steve Jamison. *Wooden on Leadership*. New York: McGraw-Hill, 2005, 302.

ABOUT THE AUTHOR

Dr. Gerald S. Levey, a nationally recognized leader in both academic medicine and private sector medical affairs, was vice chancellor, Medical Sciences and dean of the David Geffen School of Medicine from 1996 to 2010. He is presently dean emeritus and the Lincy Foundation Distinguished Service Chair. He holds the academic rank of Distinguished Professor of Medicine in the Department of Medicine. As vice chancellor, Medical Sciences at UCLA, he oversaw a diverse medical enterprise including the David Geffen School of Medicine at UCLA, the Ronald Reagan UCLA Medical Center, the Stewart and Lynda Resnick UCLA Neuropsychiatric Hospital, the Mattel Children's Hospital and Santa Monica/UCLA Medical Center and Orthopaedic Hospital.

Dr. Levey joined UCLA in September 1994, having previously served as senior vice president for medical and scientific affairs at Merck & Co., one of the world's leading pharmaceutical companies. He has held major leadership positions throughout his career, including serving as chair of the Department of Medicine at the University of Pittsburgh School of Medicine from 1979 to 1991. He is past president of the Association of Professors of Medicine, was a member of the Board of Governors of the American Board of Internal Medicine and is a member of the Association of American Physicians. Dr. Levey is also a member of the medical honorary society Alpha Omega Alpha, and is a recipient of the Distinguished Alumnus Award from the University of Medicine and Dentistry of New Jersey. He received his Mastership from the American College of Physicians in 1997.

Dr. Levey is an internist and endocrinologist widely known for his research on the thyroid gland and the heart. He was named a Howard Hughes Medical Institute Investigator while at the University of Miami from 1971 to 1979. Dr. Levey has developed a particular interest in issues of the nation's physician supply and the role of generalist physicians, and served as co-chair of the National Study of Internal Medicine Manpower from 1981 to 1991. He has authored or co-authored 210 scientific publications. Among his honors he is the recipient of the UCLA Medal (the highest award given by UCLA); The Award of Extraordinary Merit, UCLA Medical Alumni Association; Charles Drew University of Medicine and Science Board Medal of Honor; The American Jewish Committee Distinguished Leadership Award; Gerald S. Levey Surgical Award, UCLA Department of Surgery; Visionary Award, UCLA Department of Neurosurgery; The Golden Apple Award, David Geffen School of Medicine Class of 2010; Barbara A. Levey, MD and Gerald S. Levey, MD Endowed Chair donated by Robert A. (Bobby) and Nina Kotick; and Gerald S. Levey, MD Endowed Chair, donated by Shirley and Ralph Shapiro.